Donor Insemination: International Social Science Perspectives

Donor insemination or DI is the oldest and most widely practised form of assisted conception. Until now, it has largely been assessed as if an entirely medical concern. This book brings together an international group of social scientists to discuss the social, cultural, political and practical dimensions to DI, relating it to the wider debates about fertility treatment and the place of assisted conception in contemporary society. The contributors consider the experience of DI from the viewpoints of all the various parties involved, including the recipients of the treatment, the sperm providers, the clinicians, the people conceived and policy-makers working in the area. The assumptions informing the world-wide practices around DI and the reactions to it are critically examined, with reference to cross-national perspectives, and to issues such as the language of DI, gender, sexuality, ethnicity and identity.

KEN DANIELS is Associate Professor in the Department of Social Work, at the University of Canterbury, Christchurch, New Zealand. He has written widely on the policy issues and psychosocial aspects of assisted conception, and is a member of the New Zealand National Ethics committee on Assisted Human Reproduction.

ERICA HAIMES is Senior Lecturer in Sociology in the Department of Social Policy, at the University of Newcastle, in England. She has written extensively on the issues concerning families and identities raised by forms of assisted conception, and is co-author (with Noel Timms) of *Adoption, identity and social policy*.

T0381755

Donor Insemination
International Social Science
Perspectives

Edited by

Ken Daniels and Erica Haimes

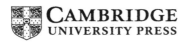

CAMBRIDGE
UNIVERSITY PRESS

CAMBRIDGE UNIVERSITY PRESS
Cambridge, New York, Melbourne, Madrid, Cape Town,
Singapore, São Paulo, Delhi, Tokyo, Mexico City

Cambridge University Press
The Edinburgh Building, Cambridge CB2 8RU, UK

Published in the United States of America by Cambridge University Press, New York

www.cambridge.org
Information on this title: www.cambridge.org/9780521497831

© Cambridge University Press 1998

First published 1998

A catalogue record for this publication is available from the British Library

ISBN 978-0-521-49709-1 Hardback
ISBN 978-0-521-49783-1 Paperback

KD: To Tricia for her love, unstinting support and many sacrifices

EH: To my family, friends and Robin to thank them for all their love and support.

Contents

Figures

Tables

Notes on contributors

ROBERT H. BLANK is Professor of Political Science at the University of Canterbury, Christchurch, New Zealand. He is author of numerous articles and books on biomedical policy including *Rationing medicine* (1988), *Regulating reproduction* (1990), *The politics of pregnancy* (1994), and *Human reproduction, emerging technologies, and conflicting rights* (1995).

KEN DANIELS is Associate Professor in the Department of Social Work at the University of Canterbury in Christchurch, New Zealand. He has been working in the field of assisted conception and particularly DI for twenty years, and during that time has published over sixty papers. He has been used as a consultant by government or government appointed bodies in the United Kingdom, the United States, Canada, Sweden, Australia and New Zealand.

JEANETTE EDWARDS is a lecturer in social anthropology at the University of Keele. She has carried out anthropological research in the north of England in both community and organisational settings. She is co-author of *Technologies of procreation: kinship in the age of assisted conception* (1993) and is presently completing *Born and Bred: Ideas of Relatedness and Relationships in Late-Twentieth-Century England*, addressing contemporary understandings of new reproductive technologies, based on fieldwork in the north west of England.

ERICA HAIMES is Senior Lecturer in Sociology, in the Department of Social Policy, University of Newcastle upon Tyne, United Kingdom. She has been working in the areas of health, adoption and assisted conception for fifteen years. Her doctoral thesis was entitled 'Family Connections: The Management of Biological Origins in the New Reproductive Technologies'; she is co-author (with Noel Timms) of *Adoption, identity and social policy* (Gower) and she is currently working on another book provisionally titled "Families and Identities".

JUDITH LASKER is NEH Distinguished Professor and Chair of the Department of Sociology and Anthropology at Lehigh University in Bethlehem, Pennsylvania, United States. She received her PhD in sociology from Harvard in 1976. She is co-author with Susan Borg of two books: *When pregnancy fails: families coping with miscarriage, ectopic pregnancy, stillbirth, and infant death* and *In search of parenthood: coping with infertility and high tech conception*. Her research and teaching interests focus on women's health, bereavement, infertility and AIDS.

SIMONE BATEMAN NOVAES is a sociologist and full-time researcher at the Centre de Recherche Sens, Ethique et Société (CERSES) of the Centre National de la Recherche Scientifique (CNRS) in Paris, France. Her research focuses on ethical questions raised by novel medical practices, particularly in the area of reproduction, as well as on the legal and political aspects of these issues. She is interested in the way social practices are constructed around technical innovations which question our usual conceptions of being and acting human. She has recently published *Les passeurs de gametes* and has edited a volume *Biomedicine et devenir de la personne* (1991).

ELIZABETH SNOWDEN is a Research Fellow in the Sociology Department, Exeter University. Together with Robert Snowden she is conducting a long-term, prospective, follow-up study of couples who are parents of children conceived by donor insemination. She is a founder-member of the British Infertility Counselling Association and an Honorary Life Member of the Family Planning Association. She has lectured and published widely on the social implications of the new reproductive technologies.

ROBERT SNOWDEN is the Professor of Family Studies in the Sociology Department, Exeter University. During the last twenty-five years his research interests have focused exclusively on the topic of reproductive behaviour. The research institute he founded in Exeter University is designated a Collaborating Centre for Research in Human Reproduction by the World Health Organisation. He was a founder-member of the Human Fertilisation and Embryology Authority (1990-1993) and is an Honorary Life Member of the Family Planning Association. In 1994, he was admitted as a Fellow of the Faculty of Family Planning and Reproductive Health Care of the Royal College of Obstetricians and Gynaecologists. Robert and Elizabeth Snowden are among the first to have undertaken research into the social and personal implications of donor insemination.

Acknowledgements

We wish to acknowledge the financial support provided by the University of Newcastle, UK. Senior Visiting Fellowship Fund and the Department of Social Policy Research Fund and by the University of Canterbury Research Fund. Our thanks to Marilyn Strathern, Meg Stacey, Robyn Rowland, Rona Achilles and Bob Snowden who have all in different ways contributed to our thinking. A very grateful thank you to Yvette Haimes, Dorothy McLoughlin, Barbara Seaton, Rosalie Kennedy and Maureen Woods for their assistance in preparing the manuscript. A special thanks to Catherine Max and her colleagues for their support and guidance.

List of abbreviations

AFS	American Fertility Society
AHR	assisted human reproduction
AI	artificial insemination
AID	artificial insemination by donor
AIDS	Acquired Immune Deficiency Syndrome
AIH	artificial insemination by husband
ART	assisted reproductive technologies
BAAF	British Agencies for Adoption and Fostering
CECOS	Centre d'Etude et Conservation du Sperme (and more recently, Centre d'Etude et de Conservation des Oeufs et du Sperme Humaine)
DI	donor insemination
GIFT	gamete intra-fallopian transfer
HFE Act (1990)	Human Fertilisation and Embryology Act, United Kingdom (1990)
HFEA	Human Fertilisation and Embryology Authority, United Kingdom
HIV	human immunodeficiency virus
ICSI	intra cytoplasmic sperm injection
IVF	*in vitro* fertilization
NAC	National Association for the Childless, United Kingdom
OTA	Office of Technology Assessment, United States Congress
RCNRT	Canadian Royal Commission on New Reproductive Technologies
RCOG	Royal College of Obstetricians and Gynaecologists, United Kingdom

1 International social science perspectives on donor insemination: an introduction

Erica Haimes and Ken Daniels

In this book we aim to present the first systematic social science analysis of donor insemination (DI): the process through which a (usually anonymous) fertile man provides semen (most often with the assistance of medical personnel) to a fertile women in order to help her try to conceive a child. The major indication for the use of DI is that the female does not have a fully fertile male partner. We also aim to locate this practice in its global setting. In pursuing these aims we shall be both documenting, and contributing to, the debates on practice and policy around DI that have emerged in the latter half of the twentieth century and that promise to shape the social identity of DI in the first part of the next century.

It is especially appropriate to tackle this task now since donor insemination has been practised for just over 100 years (the first successful case occurred in 1884) and is the oldest technique in 'the new technologies of reproduction'. DI has remained hidden from public view and scrutiny for much of that time, only emerging fully on to the public agenda with the development, in the 1970s and 1980s, of other related technologies of reproduction, such as *in vitro* fertilisation and egg donation. There are numerous strands to the historical development, and current social context of DI, both as a medical technique and as a solution to the problem of infertility: these require identification and disentangling. In this book we make a start on that task by presenting an analysis that focuses on the perspectives on DI from a range of social groups involved: the users of DI; the semen providers; the clinicians; the policy makers; the wider community. The major theme that recurs throughout these different perspectives is the analysis of why DI has been hidden from such scrutiny for so long and what impact that secrecy has had on all parties involved, as well as on DI as a social practice. Clearly these perspectives overlap with and inform each other. In documenting the nature of these overlapping influences we, as social scientists, can begin to gain analytical purchase on the complex web of social relationships that DI both reflects and constitutes as part of a wider social order.

For the sake of clarity we shall briefly outline here what the practice of DI can involve but, in so doing, we note that any such description itself

1

constructs the practice of DI in a particular, perspectival way. Thus, we shall merely sketch out the possible outlines that give it some shape: some of the following chapters will colour those in, whilst others will provide alternative sketches which render DI a rather different shape and colouring. It is the claim of this collection that such variations are, paradoxically, the essence of DI and, of course, of social life as a whole.

Donor insemination emerged from the medical problem of infertility. The first account of a successful insemination using donated semen was published in 1909, but described events in 1884, when the sperm from 'the best looking member' of a doctor's class was used to inseminate a merchant's wife, who successfully conceived. Neither she nor her husband knew what had taken place though the doctor did tell the husband when he heard of the pregnancy. At the husband's request the wife was never told. The author of this article reports shaking the hand of the twenty five year old, in 1909; the reader is left to assume that the author was also the sperm provider (Achilles 1992: 15–16).

Donor insemination does not cure male infertility but rather provides a way of circumventing the associated difficulties. Uses of DI have expanded in the late twentieth century to situations where a male partner carries a genetic disorder and thus where the use of donor semen can avoid the onward transmission of that disorder, or where a male partner has had a vasectomy, or where a woman wishes for a child but has no male partner or wishes to avoid intercourse with a man.

Thus, from a clinical point of view, the issues around DI concern questions of diagnosis, treatment, how and when to suggest DI, success rates, how to recruit semen donors and how to mediate the relationship between recipients of DI and the providers of donated semen. The only accurate figures available regarding the use of DI emanate from Britain and France. While other countries, most notably Australia, New Zealand, the United States, collect data on assisted human reproduction (AHR) technologies, DI is not included. In 1994 in the United Kingdom a total of 8,096 women received 21,180 cycles of treatment and this resulted in the birth of 1,805 children (HFEA 1996). Alnot (1993) says that 20,525 cycles of DI were carried out in France in 1991 resulting in the birth of 1,777 children. A United States Report (OTA 1988) estimated that 86,000 cycles of treatment were provided resulting in the birth of 33,000 children.

However, since the purpose of DI is to create a baby, another way of looking at the practice (as evidenced by the 1909 report mentioned above) is to describe it in terms of making and becoming parents, of having children and forming families. Such a reformulation makes it explicit that DI is about social relationships and social processes that incorporate, but also go beyond, the medical perspective. This raises additional questions. Who is making the decisions about the use of DI? Who is actually making these parents? What types of children are being conceived? What types of families are being made? What types of donors are being used? It is not that clinicians are unaware of these other questions, it is just that they are confronted on a day to day basis with other, more immediate questions of practice and practicality. It is the social scientist's task to ask these other questions and to analyse their significance to the wider socio-cultural context. That is what the authors in this collection are doing: asking about, documenting and analysing the social relationships that shape and change both the development and deployment of DI as a social as well as a clinical practice.

In claiming that this book presents a social science perspective we have the following points in mind. First, we follow Giddens in the view that the social science endeavour is multidisciplinary, involving the combination of the 'sociological imagination', with 'historical sensibility' and 'anthropological insight' (1982: 22). We would also add social psychology to that list as a means of addressing the language of individual behaviour and motivation. Secondly, such an approach enables us to address questions concerning DI at the level of the conceptual, the empirical, the cultural, the political and the practical (Stacey 1992). The purpose of such a multi-layered approach is that it enables the contributors to this volume to address issues surrounding, and the reactions to, donor insemination. Thirdly, the social science approach has itself to be reflective: to acknowledge, that is, the provisional basis of its own claims. Far from being a weakness this allows the possibility of dialogue and inter-connections between our social science approach and that of other disciplines (e.g. medicine and science) and between the apparently narrow issues of donor insemination and the wider field of social life.

This also explains why it is so important to take a global perspective on these issues. Since the practice of, and market for, DI is worldwide, it is only by knowing about what is going on in a range of countries that one can begin to participate in a fully informed dialogue. One needs to be able to document the similarities and differences in practice between different countries in order to break free from familiar patterns of thought and to be able to place these comparisons in their cultural, conceptual, empirical, political and practical contexts. Thus, this collection has authors from the United States, the United Kingdom, France and New Zealand, who each draw upon their extensive research knowledge of Canada, Australia, Scandinavia, eastern and southern Europe and Latin America.

Thus the notion of dialogue comes to the fore again. We hope that this book will contribute to and provoke further dialogues around the world on DI from a number of different perspectives, since this collection represents the thinking of leading social scientists who are working in and writing about this area. In chapter 2, Judith Lasker explores the issues that arise for the users of DI, as they go through the process of considering, and then deciding to use, DI. She describes their assessment of the costs, the risks and the alternatives to DI use. She also analyses how they perceive the man who provides the semen and their concerns for the child who is conceived from this donated semen. In her analysis she draws out the similarities and differences between the various user groups, including heterosexual couples, single women and lesbian couples.

In chapter 3, Robert and Elizabeth Snowden build upon their pioneering work in the field of DI in the 1970s to explore the issues that arise for the families that are created through the use of DI. Using data taken primarily from their own interviews with parents, the Snowdens analyse the nature of biological and nurturing family relationships and of how their, and our, understanding and experience of these has been shaped by DI. One theme around which other aspects of these relationships turn is the question of how much information about the child's conception is shared within the family. The Snowdens demonstrate, through rich and detailed data, that, whether they decide to tell their child or not, this is an aspect that no DI parents can ignore.

In chapter 4, Erica Haimes suggests that one of the legacies of not telling children about their DI conception is that we have very little data on how people who have been conceived in this way view that fact. What we have instead is very full data on how others have claimed the authority to speak on their behalf. Haimes explores the historical and social processes through which those claims have been established and the ways in which these claims have led to certain characterisations of the people conceived as having par-ticular needs and interests. The emerging body of data that directly presents the views of the people conceived, although still thin, provides a potential challenge to these characterisations and thus to policy and practice.

In chapter 5 Ken Daniels uses a historical perspective to show how the position of the semen provider has moved from one of obscurity to one of acknowledgment. He argues that the next stage needs to be one of valuing the semen provider for the contribution he makes, especially when that contribution is analysed in terms of gift dynamics and when efforts are made to reduce the marginalisation of providers. Daniels' worldwide review of research also indicates that semen providers have rather more complex motivations and views than they have commonly been attributed with by the clinicians who have usually spoken on their behalf. This research also indicates that semen providers are more open to the possibility of future contact with offspring than had previously been assumed.

The chapter by Simone Novaes highlights how DI came to be con-structed as a medical treatment for male infertility, through the focus on DI as merely a technical act under clinical management. Thus the doctor came to fulfil a mediating role between the infertile couple and the semen provider which, in turn, allowed for the establishment and maintenance of secrecy between recipients and providers. The advent of semen banks moved DI from its quasi-clandestine position to one of greater social acceptance. Novaes concludes her chapter by asking questions about the extent to which the specific domain of competence that clinicians inhabit legitimises their role in making wider decisions about reproduction.

Robert Blank shifts the focus to the public policy context and asks what role, if any, governments ought to play in regulating fertility services, and reproduction more generally. He explores the regulatory options that are available to cover the DI field and cautions against 'excessive public control'. He provides a worldwide overview of the current regulation covering DI in different countries, highlighting the diversity of approaches adopted but also highlighting the number of areas in which no regulation exists. He suggests the UK Human Fertilisation and Embryology Authority provides one regulatory model that has 'promise' and argues that an approach is needed that provides a form of public accountability.

In the final substantive chapter, Jeanette Edwards, an anthropologist, examines the question of whether we can usefully talk about 'public opinion' in relation to DI. In exploring the views held by people not directly involved in DI she notes that most made sense of this procedure in terms of its potential for creating and affecting social relationships. The people with whom Edwards discussed these issues drew upon their own experiences of kinship to make sense of DI and were able to turn the issues around and see them from a range of different perspectives: at one point from the child's perspective, at another point from the recipients' perspective. This not only alerts us to the dangers of assuming that any one individual can only speak from one perspective, it also alerts us to the dangers of assuming that there is only one 'public' and only one 'opinion'.

In the concluding chapter we return to the theme of the multiplicity of perspectives in order to reflect on those which have been most influential in directing our thinking about DI and those which have, until recently, been relatively neglected. We consider a range of debates that have yet to be conducted around DI whilst, at the same time, noting just how much the authors in this collection have helped to broaden the existing analysis of donor insemination.

REFERENCES

Alnot, M. (1993) '1992 results of sperm donor procreation. French Federation of CECOS and private cooperative centers'. *Contraception, Fertilité, Sexualité* 21(5): 371:3.

Achilles, R. (1992) *Donor insemination: an overview.* Royal Commission on New Reproductive Technologies, Ontario, Canada.

Giddens, A. (1982) *Sociology: a brief, but critical introduction.* London: Macmillan.

Human Fertilisation and Embryology Authority (1996). *Fifth Annual Report 1996.*

Stacey, M. ed. (1992) *Changing human reproduction: social science perspectives.* London: Sage.

United States Congress. Office of Technology Assessment. (1988) *Infertility: medical and social choices,* Washington DC: US Government Printing Office.

2   The users of donor insemination

Judith N. Lasker

Introduction

Donor insemination (DI) is the oldest, most widely used, and probably most effective alternative method of conception in use today. Yet its use continues to be fraught with anxieties, controversies, and a deep cloak of secrecy. Those who consider donor insemination often do so at first with great reluctance and with fears about the ramifications and the results. The focus of this chapter is on the concerns and experiences of those who are potential or actual users of DI. Donor insemination has two very distinct types of users, and these two groups have almost entirely different needs and priorities, different experiences and different dilemmas. Although most fertility programmes are geared exclusively or primarily to married couples, and in some countries they are limited by law to married couples, donor insemination is increasingly being used in many parts of the world by single women, both heterosexual and lesbian. Two important changes are pushing this trend: alternative treatments have become increasingly available that allow men with severe fertility impairments to father children, eliminating the need for a donor, and the idea of single motherhood through insemination has become more widely accepted. In addition, the possibility of finding ones own donor and carrying out the insemination at home eliminates for many single women the necessity of having to get past the barriers that exist to their using medical services (Stephenson and Wagner 1991). Thus, there is reason to believe that single women are gaining rapidly in their representation among insemination clients (Leiblum *et al.* 1995).

Many single women, both lesbian and heterosexual, consider it to be an important advantage that they can conceive a wanted child without concern about sexual and emotional involvement with a man and without the stigma which may be associated with becoming pregnant accidentally. Donor insemination allows them to explain to the children, and to others, that this was a planned and desired conception, and it allows them to select desired characteristics of the genetic father and to have some confidence that he has been screened for genetic and other illness.

For heterosexual couples in which the man is infertile, donor insemination offers the possibility of having an apparently 'normal' pregnancy and birth with the man present at both the conception and birth. Both partners can share the experience of pregnancy just like any fertile couple, without ever having to reveal the man's infertility. In contrast to adoption, the child will have a genetic tie to one member of the couple, and there will not be the uncertainty about the physical and social conditions in which the birth mother carried the pregnancy.

Donor insemination is also the simplest and least expensive form of alternative conception. Because of the apparent disadvantages and the growing difficulties and higher costs associated with adoption, insemination has become increasingly popular among many couples in which the man is infertile as well as among lesbians and single heterosexual women. Occasionally, donor insemination is chosen by couples in which the man carries a genetic trait which they do not want to pass along to the child, or where both members carry a recessive gene which may result in a child having a serious illness. It is also used in cases where the male partner had a vasectomy or has undergone chemotherapy. There have been a few cases of widows using the sperm of their deceased husbands; in one case a woman asked for sperm to be withdrawn shortly after her husband's sudden and violent death (Caplan 1995).

Although technically quite simple and in use for many years (it is therefore inaccurate on at least two counts to call donor insemination a 'new reproductive technology'), there are serious social and psychological issues which emerge from the use of DI. This chapter will focus on the experiences of men and women who consider and try DI and on the types of issues and dilemmas which they face. In particular, I will consider what is known about: first, the decision to try DI; second, the effects of going through the procedure; and third, the looming issue of secrecy. Many of these issues affect the two client groups quite differently. Therefore, in discussing each of the three subjects, I will first address the common concerns of both groups and then consider the concerns which are particular to each group separately.

Much of the information and all of the quotations used in this chapter come from a study of people who considered or tried various methods of achieving pregnancy (Lasker and Borg 1994). Respondents were recruited by word of mouth, through infertility clinics, and by notices in the newsletters of the RESOLVE infertility support group. Approximately two dozen subjects were interviewed by phone, and the interviews were taped (with permission) and transcribed. An additional ninety-four people completed questionnaires sent out to those who responded to the request in RESOLVE newsletters. Thus, as in most studies, they do not represent all infertile people or all people using artificial means of conception, but rather they reflect many of the concerns and opinions of people who are able to consider using these methods and are willing to talk about their experiences. Findings from this study are combined in this chapter with results from the work of others who have studied programmes of donor insemination and the people who use them.

Considering donor insemination

The possibility of donor insemination begins for the majority of heterosexual couples when they recognize that the man is unable to produce sufficient numbers of healthy sperm to fertilise the woman's eggs *in vivo*. Thus the first and most important issue to be faced is the reality of his infertility. For single women, infertility is rarely the reason for choosing DI. For them, it is a very different recognition, that they are not going to have a male partner with whom to conceive a child. This may be by choice in the case of lesbians, who often have committed women partners, or by 'default' in the case of heterosexual women who have not found a suitable partner or do not want one and do not want to wait any longer to become mothers.

Issues for both groups. Both groups have to consider the costs in time, money, and stress of going through the procedure, the chances of success and the physical risks, as well as their feelings about using a donor. Both may also have concerns about the effects of using DI on their relationships and on any future children, but these will be addressed separately for the two groups.

1. *Cost.* The costs of the procedure are part of the challenge. Although artificial insemination usually costs far less than *in vitro* fertilisation or hiring a surrogate mother, the monthly expenses mount up quickly. Each time a woman is inseminated, there is the charge for the office visit and the fee for the sperm sample. In addition, she may be taking expensive fertility drugs to stimulate her ovulation. The American Office of Technology Assessment's 1987 survey of practitioners of artificial insemination concluded that the average patient cost for four cycles was about $1,000, with physicians who carry out the most inseminations reporting considerably higher charges. Approximately three-fourths of the total costs in the United States are paid by the patients themselves (Office of Technology Assessment 1988). A recent report gave much higher estimates: that an initial work-up costs between $400 and $500, and each cycle can cost anywhere from $500 to $2,500 depending on the technology used ('Sperm Banks and Clinics' 1994).

There is also a non-monetary cost, such as the pressures of checking daily temperatures and being available for insemination at the time of ovulation.

There is often a great deal of inconvenience, compounded by the anxiety and stress of the procedure. Women who have been through DI often complain about the difficulty of coordinating their ovulation with the physician's schedule. The increased use of frozen sperm has alleviated the logistics problems somewhat, as it is no longer necessary in these cases to coordinate with the donor as well.

2. *Risks*. Donor insemination increasingly involves treatment of the woman with powerful drugs. In the last few years, many fertility centres have introduced the use of superovulation through hormonal treatment of the woman before insemination because of the greater likelihood of pregnancy after hormone injections. Nevertheless, these drugs are inconvenient to administer, expensive, and often have side effects (Stephenson and Wagner 1993).

Another risk of donor insemination is the possibility of transmitting infections or genetic disorders. A study of 316 Danish and Swedish couples who had been through DI revealed that 85 per cent of them had worried about contracting a sexually transmitted disease as a result of donor insemination (Nielsen *et al.* 1995). A recent study identified seven cases of women in five fertility clinics in the United States and Canada who were infected with HIV through DI prior to 1986; while the availability of screening has greatly reduced this risk, it remains a concern for many women (Araneta *et al.* 1995).

3. *Success rates*. Studies of donor insemination report widely varying success rates, dependent in part on the woman's age and the treatment strategy. Generally DI is much more likely than IVF to result in pregnancy, but many couples are surprised that it may take six months or longer of inseminations before this may be accomplished, and some drop out after one or more attempts.

4. *The donor*. Perhaps the greatest concern of those who are deciding whether or not to try DI is over the identity, the health, and the characteristics of the donor. Usually the donor is not known to the couple at all unless they seek him out themselves. In most cases, the physician finds a donor, either through personal contacts or through a sperm bank, and the identity is carefully guarded. Baran and Pannor (1989) found that many couples fantasise about the donor and have considerable anxiety about him.

Many people who use DI express uncertainty about the real identity and characteristics of the donor. One woman commented: 'They asked what characteristics we wanted from the donor but warned that special requests might mean a delay since there were so few donors. We often joked that it was probably one guy who went behind a screen and put on a different wig each time depending upon the request'.

Such joking reflects considerable anxiety on the part of many couples about the donor's identity. News events about unusual cases can certainly contribute to this anxiety. For example, several couples reported that they had experienced worries during the pregnancy about a racial mix-up (Lasker and Borg 1994). In June 1995, it was reported that just such an error had occurred in a Dutch fertility clinic, with a couple undergoing IVF having twins, one darker than the other, because sperm from an Aruban man was left in the pipette in which the Dutch man's semen was placed to fertilise his wife's ova (Simons 1995).

Speculation and concern about the appearance of the donor are common among people going through DI and in particular during a pregnancy resulting from insemination. A study of Polish couples seeking DI found some of them wanting more information about the characteristics of the donor, and most of them were concerned that he should look like the husband (Bielawska-Batorowicz 1994). Of 316 Danish couples who had been through DI, 82 per cent agreed that before the treatment, they had speculated about the appearance of the donor and whether the child would look like them; a third wished they had more descriptive information about the donor (Nielsen *et al.* 1995). The same desire for more information was expressed by single heterosexual and lesbian women in an American study; in this study, the donor characteristics of greatest importance to the women were education, ethnicity, and height (Leiblum *et al.* 1995).

Some women also worry that the doctor might himself be the donor. Accounts of the physician being the donor are indeed nothing new. There was a great deal of publicity in the United States about the arrest and conviction of an American physician who had used his own semen in many cases without informing the patients (Snowden *et al.* 1983; Rubin 1995).

People who have used donor insemination report widely differing feelings toward the donor. Some wish they could meet him and see what he looks like or thank him for his help. Others dismiss the donor, saying they have purchased a product and the person producing it is irrelevant to them. Most people know that they will never be able to find out who the donor is and prefer to try to forget about him. Some fathers are plagued by feelings of inferiority when they compare themselves to the bright and accomplished type of man who is selected to be a donor (Lasker and Borg 1994; Baran and Pannor 1989).

Because of the potential problems with choosing donors, some couples and many single women decide to select their own and avoid physicians altogether. Another reason for this results from new policies which encourage the use of frozen sperm due to concerns about the transmission of disease, and in particular of HIV infection. When semen is frozen, the donor can be screened for HIV both at the time of the donation and again six months later before the specimen is used. Frozen semen is, however, more expensive and has a lower success rate, thus often requiring additional cycles before pregnancy is achieved (Barlet and Penney 1994; Nachtigall 1994). As a result, some potential users of DI seek out their own donor and try to avoid the sperm banks. A relative of the husband or a close friend may be asked. The majority of people, however, prefer not to know the donor because of anticipated complications in their relationships, or else they cannot find a willing man, and thus they rely on the uncertainty but also the anonymity of a donor programme.

Heterosexual couples

Heterosexual couples thinking about using donor insemination must consider some specific issues, including the alternatives available to them, the impact of male partner infertility and of DI on their relationship, and concerns about the effect on future children. These issues differ to some extent depending on the reasons why DI may be selected.

1. *Reasons for considering DI*. Most heterosexual couples choose DI for one of three reasons: infertility, prior vasectomy, or to avoid transmitting an unwanted genetic trait. Yet there have been almost no studies of how these differences affect the experience of DI or the choice to use it.

One exception is the study by Baran and Pannor (1989), who interviewed individuals and couples who used DI for all three reasons mentioned above. Their sample included twelve men and thirty women in couples where the husband was infertile, thirteen men and seven women who used DI because of a vasectomy, and four couples in which the man had a genetic problem he did not want to pass along to his children. They were recruited primarily through newspaper ads and were almost all middle to upper-middle class. They found striking differences between the people who used DI for infertility and the other two groups. The infertile men were much more uncomfortable about using DI and were more likely to feel inadequate and powerless in their families. They were also the most concerned about keeping DI secret. In many cases they were convinced by the physician and by their wives to resort to DI just after learning of their infertility and thus had no opportunity to grieve the loss or deal with the shock. DI was seen by others as a 'solution' but was accepted by the men only with a great deal of anguish and ambivalence. In contrast, the men who had genetic problems were not concerned about their infertility and had come to the decision not to father children on their own, sometimes before getting married. They were the most comfortable with the idea of donor insemination, and in the case which Baran and Pannor describe, insisted on meeting the donor father and on telling the children of their origins.

In the middle, but most like the second group, were men who had had vasectomies and had had children before. They had proven their fertility and were not concerned about their masculinity. They tended to regret having had the vasectomy, but their biggest concern was about becoming parents again, often at an age when they already had grown children. Yet Baran and Pannor report that they were often the most relaxed about parenting and enjoyed their new children with a minimum of stress. This is consistent with the findings of Humphrey and Humphrey (1993), who studied men who had had vasectomies and then had children with DI. The authors suggest that these men tend to be older and to have had children in a previous marriage, and that as a result they are more mature and more sensitive to their wives' desire for children.

2. *Alternatives.* Couples in which the man is infertile have for years had to choose between adoption, DI, and not having children. In recent years, they have had another option due to the increased use of *in vitro* fertilisation for male infertility and in particular the development of a variety of techniques for micromanipulation of sperm, which introduce sperm directly into the egg in a laboratory. These developments allow men who have a very low sperm count the possibility of fertilising ova in IVF programmes. Until the development of micromanipulation techniques, such as ICSI (intra cytoplasmic sperm injection), the possibilities of fertilisation were very low when the man was oligospermic. Today there is a chance that the woman's eggs can be successfully fertilised with only a few sperm through IVF procedures (Ben-Chetrit *et al*. 1995; Tucker 1995; Palermo *et al*. 1995). This procedure, when compared to DI, is much more expensive, involves more physical risks for the woman, and has a lower success rate. Yet some couples are willing to attempt it, and many infertility specialists are sure to recommend it instead of DI, in order for the man to have a genetic tie to the child and to avoid the difficulties posed by having a donor.

As new techniques for dealing with male infertility improve and become more widely available outside major medical centres in a limited number of countries, the demand for donor insemination by heterosexual couples is certain to drop. Those who choose DI over IVF are likely to do so because of the unavailability, inconvenience or cost of the latter, or after failing to achieve a pregnancy with IVF.

Most couples who choose DI consider adoption first, and some actually begin adoption proceedings. In Daniels' study (1994) of fifty-four couples in New Zealand who gave birth after DI, 72 per cent had considered or attempted adoption. They ended up choosing DI both because of the advantage it offered for the woman to have a genetic and biological tie to the child and also because of the uncertainties and difficulties presented by adoption. Owens and colleagues (1993) mailed questionnaires to approximately 500 couples who belonged to the British National Association for the Childless and who were listed in the NAC records as having infertility attributed to the male partner. This is clearly a quite atypical group, but useful in the findings obtained. Analysis of 205 useable responses showed that, while 32 per cent were considering adoption and 41 per cent had taken active steps in that direction or had already adopted a child, two-thirds of the sample still indicated that they felt that DI was the only way of overcoming infertility. Indeed, 61 per cent of the sample had taken active steps toward DI, and the majority of those had already conceived or become parents. Approximately a fifth of the sample was also considering IVF or GIFT, and another 23 per cent had taken active steps in that direction.

In a Danish study of couples who had tried DI, 23 per cent said they had first tried to adopt a child; the remainder said they preferred to have a biological link and therefore had rejected adoption (Rosenkvist 1981). A Polish study of thirty-five couples who had sought donor insemination also found that they had concluded that DI would be preferable to adoption (Bielawska-Batorowicz 1994).

It would be very useful to have a comparable study of couples who considered DI and then rejected it in favour of adoption. One reason given in the study of RESOLVE members (Lasker and Borg 1994) by couples rejecting DI in favour of adoption was that they preferred to have no biological connection to the child rather than to have an unequal one in which only one parent would be connected genetically. In the Owens study (1993), those couples who had rejected DI gave as the most frequent reason (43 per cent) their discomfort with a third party being the genetic father and the likelihood of deception associated with that fact. The second most frequently given reason related to ethical or religious concerns. Also mentioned by some couples was preference for adoption or IVF, worry about marital problems arising from DI, hope that a natural pregnancy would still be possible, and the fear of AIDS. Some of these couples who rejected DI indicated that they would be willing to reconsider if other means did not work.

3. *Relationship issues.* Couples who consider DI for infertility follow a somewhat different trajectory from those who are considering IVF or other routes to pregnancy. In these other cases the woman is extensively tested and treated, and the cause of infertility is sought in her body. Even when both partners are found to have fertility impairments, the majority of testing and treatment is carried out on the woman. The major difference with DI is that it is appropriate for couples in which the woman is at least relatively fertile and the man is completely or almost completely lacking in sperm. Thus the cultural assumption of infertility being primarily a female problem is violated for these couples.

For the man, there is often a blow to his sense of himself as a man if he is infertile. Some men feel ashamed that they cannot father a child; others feel that they have let their wives down. Some are upset that they cannot pass the family genes on to the next generation. For the woman, there may be anger at her partner, guilt for feeling angry, and guilt that she is fertile when he is not. With both husband and wife feeling angry with themselves and with each other, it is not surprising that conflict may develop between them. Thus couples considering DI often wonder about the possible effects of going through the procedure and of a subsequent birth on their relationship.

Researchers have concluded that women generally appear to be more distressed and preoccupied by infertility than are men (Greil *et al.* 1988; Draye *et al.* 1988; Brand 1989; Andrews *et al.* 1991). This difference in reaction may create considerable tension during the period of deciding about and then pursuing donor insemination.

Is the greater distress on the part of women equally the case when the man is infertile and the woman is not? Some researchers have concluded that the woman is more distressed regardless of which partner is infertile, while others find that both are more distressed in cases of male infertility; men tend to be more distressed by their own infertility than by that of their wives (Greil 1993). Male infertility may disrupt the unspoken assumption of the man's dominance in a relationship, giving the woman more power than either of them feels comfortable with. Some women even say they feel guilty about being 'whole' when their partners are not. There are even accounts of women ceasing to ovulate when DI begins (Reading *et al.* 1982).

In our study (Lasker and Borg 1994) we heard many reports of women who said they would cover up for their husbands' infertility, saying that the problem was their own. If they had previously told friends that the infertility was their husband's problem, and then they used DI, they would change the scenario to protect their husbands. A woman who wrote to RESOLVE expressed her bitterness about having to cover up her husband's infertility by letting others think that she was the one with a problem:

I was trying to get away from responding to infertility like a case of 'cooties', something you feel compelled to pin on 'the other guy'. So even though I knew my sexual identity was intact, it felt like a hollow reassurance. I seemed to be the only one who knew this . . . If everyone else sees you as infertile, it is hard not to react as though you are. (Hartman 1985: 3).

Another woman wrote to RESOLVE about the difficulties she was experiencing because her husband wanted no one to know that he had had a vasectomy during a previous marriage. The cover-up even affected the woman's relationship to her own mother, who felt guilty about her daughter's supposed infertility (Anonymous 1985).

Do such women who falsely assume the responsibility for infertility feel, whether consciously or unconsciously, that they are *supposed* to be the ones who are infertile, especially since that is what everyone else assumes? Does her assuming the responsibility for infertility restore the previous state of power between them?

The inequality of diagnosis often means that partners have to be very cautious in how they discuss their situation. This caution makes decision-making more complicated, sometimes leading the fertile partner to resort to subtle pressures. In one study of couples seeking donor insemination, the authors made this interesting observation:

Most often it is the husband who makes the first suggestion [to try AID], possibly because in the majority of cases the problem is felt to be particularly his. As far as the woman is concerned, she is afraid of hurting him or provoking some unexpected reaction by broaching the subject of AID ... [But] we often had the impression that the wife had done everything in her power to persuade the husband to suggest AID. (d'Elicio *et al.* 1980: 409–10)

The stresses of infertility and of decision making about treatment may affect every aspect of a couple's relationship. They may have a profound impact, for example, on a couple's sex life. The physical and emotional strain of treatment, as well as the depression which accompanies failure, often reduce interest in sex.

Utian (1983) observed, as have other researchers, that a couple's fertility problems may lead the husband or wife to have an affair. He concludes that some people may be trying to test their fertility with other partners. Infertility can affect a sexual relationship in another way. For instance, psychiatrist David Berger (1980) studied sixteen men diagnosed as having a very low or absent sperm count and discovered that eleven of them became impotent for several months following the diagnosis.

Yet Greil and colleagues (1989, 1991) note, importantly, that sexual difficulties which arise from fertility pressures and treatments do not necessarily lead to marital breakup or even to marital dissatisfaction. Couples may view their sexual problems as temporary and still find their relationship strengthened by the joint struggle to achieve a shared goal.

Researchers and practitioners who have studied the impact of insemination on couples often recommend that they wait until they have resolved their feelings about the man's infertility before starting DI (Berger 1980). Yet some have also found that infertile men are not nearly as distressed by DI as expected. Blaser and colleagues in Switzerland (1988) interviewed and administered psychological tests to four groups of men: infertile men whose wives were pregnant from DI, infertile men whose wives were still attempting DI, fertile husbands of pregnant women, and husbands who considered themselves fertile and were planning children in the future. Although they do not provide the number of subjects included in the study or how they were recruited, they conclude that the infertile men feel no more impaired or lacking in self-confidence and that they show no more symptoms of distress than the fertile men. The former indicated that they had coped well with the diagnosis and the process of insemination.

4. *Concerns about children.* There is a range of questions which heterosexual couples contemplating DI may have about their prospective children. In the forefront are their concerns about the children's' general health and genetic background, followed by whether the child will resemble them in looks and personality (Klock *et al.* 1994). In addition, many have questions about what to tell the children about their origins (see section on secrecy below) and about how the children would feel towards their father if they were to know about the DI.

Some parents also fear the consequences for their children of knowing about DI and not being able to identify their biological father. Certainly the appearance of news stories about DI children searching with great anguish for anonymous donors has given pause to some parents who wonder if they are serving children well by creating such a situation (Orenstein 1995). For some, this adds to the incentive not to tell the children; for others the conflict between wanting to be honest and knowing that such honesty may produce difficulty for the child can be a factor in choosing not to pursue DI. Again, there is very little information on this aspect of the decision-making process.

Single women

Single heterosexual and lesbian women who want very much to have children are turning more and more to DI as a solution. It has been estimated that 10,000 children conceived through DI in the United States have been born to lesbian mothers; other estimates of the number of American homosexuals who are raising children range from 1 to 2 million (McNamee 1994). The US government Office of Technology Assessment estimated that 30,000 single women undergo DI each year (1988). It is impossible to know the numbers, however, as lesbians are more likely than heterosexual single women or couples to seek out their own donors for insemination. Indeed, the total number of people using donor insemination is impossible to ascertain because of the secrecy which surrounds this procedure. This is even more the case in the countries where DI is limited by law to married women (Shenfield 1994).

The issues which single women, lesbian or heterosexual, face in deciding upon insemination are quite different from those of heterosexual couples. They have to deal with public disapproval, with lack of access to the procedure, and with legal ramifications not faced by married couples.

1. *Motivations and alternatives.* Many single heterosexual women who seek out donor insemination hope to get married but cannot wait any longer to find the right man before having children. As difficult as it is for married couples to adopt, it is even more so for unmarried women. Single heterosexual women and lesbians who are either single or in a couple have few other options besides donor insemination. Although some adoption agencies will consider single parents, the obstacles are even greater than for married couples and are particularly great for homosexuals.

Single women, straight or lesbian, may not want intimacy with a man in order to conceive, or they may prefer to avoid problems by not knowing the identity of the father (McGuire and Alexander 1985; Pies 1989; Strong and Schinfeld 1984). Among the fifteen lesbian couples in a Belgian clinic who explained why they came for DI, twelve did not want to violate their fidelity and/or sleep with a man, eight did not want to introduce a third party into their plans, eight considered it morally questionable to involve a man temporarily, and seven were afraid of being infected with HIV (Englert 1994). As one lesbian woman said, 'Sex with somebody that I'm not involved with otherwise would seem so mercenary. It wasn't anything I ever considered. I kind of liked the idea of having a virgin birth. And anyway, conception is conception, it's just a matter of how the sperm gets there'. Leiblum and colleagues (1995) surveyed fifty-one women, all of them single heterosexual and lesbian women who had completed one course of DI at a New Jersey (USA) medical school; of these, forty-five (88 per cent) responded, including twenty-eight heterosexuals, fourteen lesbians, two bisexuals and one woman who described herself as celibate. The major considerations in choosing DI for the heterosexuals, who were older than the lesbian women, were that time was running out and that they had not met a man who would be an appropriate father. The lesbians, ten of whom were living in couples, focused on wanting to share parenting with their partners and on their feeling that they had sufficient support and encouragement to embark on DI. Both groups agreed that their feelings of security in their employment and confidence that they had resolved their concerns about parenting were major factors influencing their decision to try DI.

Thus, many women who are not in a sexual relationship with a man consider donor insemination to be the best of all the alternatives for having children. Yet they also share the concerns of heterosexual couples about the identity of the donor and about the welfare of prospective children. Many of the respondents in Leiblum *et al.*'s study (1995) expressed a desire to know more personal information about the donor, such as his motives for being a donor, personality characteristics, interests, and medical background; for some of them this desire was motivated by wanting to share such information with the child.

2. *Access.* The most difficult problem faced by unmarried women is obtaining donor insemination. Many physicians and clinics refuse to inseminate anyone who is not in a stable marriage; others insist on first having a psychological evaluation (Ostrom and King 1993; Cornacchia 1994; Englert 1994). Some countries have official policies restricting donor insemination to married couples. Despite the growing number of children conceived by the artificial insemination of unmarried women, they still comprise a very small percentage of all inseminations. This proportion is certain to increase, but the obstacles, according to Stephenson and Wagner (1991), provide an example of the medical and legal professions' enforcement of social biases in relation to technologies for conception.

Public attitudes toward donor insemination, especially for single women, are changing but still unsympathetic. Many people object to DI for single or lesbian women because they believe a child born into such a situation will suffer. The British Human Fertilisation and Embryology Act of 1990 does not make it illegal to treat single women, but it does assert a 'need for a father' as a criterion for the child's welfare (Shenfield 1994). Yet studies which exist on the children of single heterosexual and lesbian mothers do not show a negative effect on children (Bleckman 1982; Strong and Schinfeld 1984; Golombok and Tasker 1994; Flaks 1995).

Other arguments against making DI available for single women include the idea that it is a treatment for male sterility and thus there is no indication for using it in situations where there is no sterility. Englert (1994) responds that DI is not a treatment for men at all; it is always a procedure performed on women and has no medical effect on infertile men.

Despite Englert's defence of DI for single women, including lesbians, the Belgian clinic with which the author is associated requires special psychological screening for such women. Interestingly, such screening is much more likely to result in turning away single heterosexual women than lesbians. In sixteen out of twenty-one requests from the former group, it was determined that the women had major family and relationship problems, with considerable trauma and sometimes abuse in their history. In these cases it was judged that the request 'seemed to be more of a desperate search for a way out of their solitude than plans for a child' (Englert 1994: 1975), and they were denied access to DI. In contrast, the fifteen lesbian women who requested DI were all in ongoing stable relationships, had substantial social and family support, and had carefully considered the implications of choosing DI. Of these, only one request was postponed while the woman sought therapy for sexual abuse in childhood (Englert 1994).

Because of the barriers, many single heterosexual and lesbian women seek out a physician or a sperm bank willing to help them, or simply to do the insemination themselves. One sperm bank in California has a large lesbian clientele and offers clients and donors the possibility of knowing each others' identities. Information regarding techniques of home insemination is widely available in networks of lesbian women seeking to avoid the difficulties (and expense) of approaching physicians.

3. *Custody*. The number of court cases over custody of children born as a result of DI is rapidly increasing. There are two main types of such cases: in one, the partner in a lesbian couple who is not the biological mother of the child either seeks to adopt the child or, if the couple separates, to have visitation rights with the child she helped to raise. The other type of case is brought by sperm donors who want more involvement with the lives of their biological children. The outcomes of such cases indicate the obstacles facing lesbian and single heterosexual mothers. Courts in several American states have ruled that even if a woman is equally involved in raising a child conceived by donor insemination, she has no legal rights to that child if she is not the biological mother (Dreyfous 1991; Selby 1995; Bailey 1995; Henry 1993). This is particularly ironic in light of the decision of the first judge in the famous 'Baby M' case, who ruled that being a biological mother gave Mary Beth Whitehead no rights at all to her child. Yet a few courts are beginning to rule in favour of the non-biological parent (McCann 1994; Dean 1994).

In a few cases, the sperm donor has won visitation rights over the objection of the lesbian or single heterosexual mother (Holding 1994). These rulings demonstrate the tremendous difference between donor insemination used by married couples and by unmarried women. In the case of a heterosexual marriage, the sperm donor has no legal rights, and the birth-mother's husband is usually considered to be the parent by law.

4. *Concerns about Children*. Many of the same concerns about the health of the child are shared by all prospective parents. For single mothers who are not in a couple, there is sometimes also anxiety about being able to take care of the child. Both lesbian and heterosexual single mothers worry that the child will be unhappy about not having a known father and that he or she will be teased or ostracised by others (Brewaeys *et al.* 1993; Curley 1995; Leiblum *et al.* 1995). Many make careful plans for how the child will be informed and how they will form networks with other similar families so that the child will not feel abnormal (Lasker and Borg 1994).

Given all of these issues, how much do we really know about the process by which people decide whether or not to try donor insemination? How many people worry over each of these concerns? How many choose not to try DI because of one or more of them? We still know very little that would allow us to answer these questions, despite the growing amount of research.

We do know that most people do not decide upon DI instantly, that they are more likely to take their time after the possibility is first raised. Klock *et al.* (1994), in their study of forty-one American couples, found that 21 per cent waited less than a month to decide, 28 per cent waited one to six months, 21 per cent waited six to twelve months, and the remaining 29 per cent started DI more than a year after diagnosis of male infertility.

Berger (1980) interviewed sixteen couples in Canada in which the man had been diagnosed as infertile from eight months to four years prior to the interview. Of the sixteen, two had decided against DI, four were still deciding, and four had pursued DI without delay. The remaining six couples had decided to try DI but had delayed from several months to several years. Those who began DI without delay were reported to be having difficulties with the process. In Owens *et al.*'s (1993) study of British couples, the average time between diagnosis and first insemination was 2.4 years, with a range from less than one month to twenty-two years.

Some of this variation reflects the fact that some men know early in life that they are sterile. But for the most part, it does indicate that the decision-making process is a challenging and difficult one, something that most people are not prepared to conclude immediately. Yet Klock *et al.* (1994) found no relationship between time taken to decide and measures of psychiatric symptomatology or marital adjustment.

Going through donor insemination

There are many stresses involved in going through donor insemination, some of which have already been mentioned with regard to deciding on whether to try it at all. The costs and pressures of the insemination, the worries about success, the anxiety about the donor: these continue and sometimes increase over time.

Some couples who have been through donor insemination now wish they had done it at home, if possible. In that way they could have avoided some of the difficulties that arise when coordinating with the physician's schedule. More important, it would have been less impersonal, and the partner could be actively involved. Some physicians teach couples how to do this if they ask for instruction.

Zoldbrod (1988) reported her findings of the experience of donor insemination, based on a study of nine women who responded to a request in newsletters of RESOLVE, the American support organisation for infertile people. These women cited eight negative feelings or problems they had experienced with insemination: lack of confidentiality in the clinic, loss of libido and sexual pleasure, loss of control in their lives related particularly to scheduling problems and errors, the inconvenience of scheduling, control struggles with the physicians, feelings of shame and humiliation during treatment, physical pain during insemination, and increased stress with the number of inseminations. Many of these problems are even more acute when the people involved are committed to keeping DI a secret; it is difficult to explain to an employer or family member why one has to disappear for a mysterious appointment periodically.

Relationship problems sometimes appear during the process of DI. A study of couples participating in donor insemination found the wives to have greater stress levels and to consider DI to be more challenging than their husbands, who focused more on the beneficial side of insemination (Prattke and Gass-Sternas 1993).

A writer who interviewed twenty-two infertile British men, whom she acknowledges to be quite unusual in their willingness to talk, found them to be less concerned about issues of sexual potency than they were with their inability to help their partner fulfil her desire for pregnancy and also a feeling of being marginalised by the process of donor insemination (Mason 1993).

Some infertility programmes offer counselling for distressed patients, but counsellors are most often used for initial screening before couples are accepted, and thus there may be a subtle pressure to deny problems. Many couples express the desire for more on-going therapeutic support as they deal with the issues surrounding donor insemination. Klock and colleagues (1994) studied forty-one couples prior to insemination and found that 95 per cent believed there should be a mandatory psychological consultation. It has even been suggested that emotional adjustment might be predictive of success in becoming pregnant, although a recent study of 120 American couples found no connection between level of distress at the time of evaluation and pregnancy outcome twenty months later. However, those identified as distressed did have one counselling session (Schover et al. 1994).

Despite some case studies that indicate psychological and relationship problems for people going through DI (Alexandre 1980; Berger 1980), larger scale research on such families has uncovered relatively few significant problems as a result. A number of studies indicate that people going through donor insemination are no more distressed and experience no greater marital difficulty than comparison groups (Klock et al. 1994; Nielsen et al. 1995). Some studies even found that couples using DI have a much lower divorce rate than average, although the validity of these results has been challenged (Milson and Bergman 1982, Humphrey and Humphrey 1987). It would appear that the divorce rate is at least no higher than among other groups and that couples consider their marriages to be the same or better than before (Levie 1967; Nielsen *et al.* 1995; Stone 1980). Perhaps the process of working through the conflicts of infertility leads to stronger relationships in those who have tried donor insemination. This issue requires much more research.

The most difficult problem for people attempting DI is often the failure to conceive. Many women assume that they will become pregnant on the first try. As with many treatments for infertility, there is usually enthusiasm on the part of the physician or clinic staff that this procedure will offer the solution that has been sought. With DI especially, the parties have been carefully screened and the timing carefully planned. When it does not work, as is most commonly the case after one attempt, many women become discouraged and depressed (Rosenkvist 1981).

Many people drop out of donor insemination after one or two cycles or even while still on a waiting list. One study of 375 couples in a New Zealand programme found 165 had withdrawn without a pregnancy. Most of these reported natural conceptions, adoption, marital separation, or moving away from the region (Danesh-Meyers *et al.* 1993). Leiblum *et al.*'s (1995) study of 45 single heterosexual and lesbian women who started DI showed that 15 per cent had stopped because it was too expensive, another 15 per cent were discouraged by the lack of success, and an additional 8 per cent dropped out because they felt it was too time-consuming or because they were not receiving support from others.

A study carried out in Ohio (USA) followed 120 couples for an average of twenty months after first requesting donor insemination. In this group, 53 per cent had become pregnant, 11 per cent never began DI, 17 per cent were continuing, and 19 per cent had dropped out. Reasons for dropping out were not given, as outcome was derived from programme files rather than interviews. Since the range of follow up was one to thirty-nine months, these data do not give an exact picture of likelihood of dropping out. None the less, the researchers discovered that the percentage of couples who either never began or dropped out early was considerably lower (17 per cent compared to 33 per cent) in the segment of their population which began after the programme hired a nurse practitioner who coordinated care and provided education and support to the couples (Schover *et al.* 1994).

Keeping donor insemination secret

Almost every discussion of donor insemination raises the question of secrecy. As with other issues addressed above, the concern for secrecy is very different depending on the DI client. For heterosexual couples, it is strongly encouraged and for the most part widely adopted. In contrast, single women are more likely to *want* the DI to be publicly known.

Heterosexual couples. Secrecy is an overriding issue at every step of the process. Because of this secrecy, donor insemination is rarely discussed, and most people are even unaware of its availability. Most physicians and other staff members of donor insemination programmes strongly encourage their patients to keep their experience of insemination a secret from everyone. They even suggest not telling the obstetrician who delivers the baby, so that the husband's name will be put on the birth certificate without hesitation. As one woman said:

> The doctor told us it's nobody else's business, that it's just between the two of us and him, and no one else has to know. That was a hard thing, you know, because so many times you want to say it. It's a hard thing to explain, and people seem to think that if you can't have your own, you shouldn't have any or you should adopt. I have a feeling his parents wouldn't accept the baby if they knew. They wouldn't think she was a part of him.

Aware of the possibility of problems, many parents wonder if they should tell a child or anyone else about the conception through DI. A recent survey of couples who had a child from DI found that 74 per cent did not intend to tell the child (Owens *et al.* 1993). This is consistent with the findings of many other studies of this topic (Bielawska-Batorowicz 1994; Ledward *et al.* 1982; Schover *et al.* 1992) although see chapter by Daniels in this collection.

It is clear that secrecy is a much greater issue with DI than with any other method of conception. In a survey of ninety-four American men and women who had considered or tried several different alternatives (Lasker and Borg 1989), those who had been through DI were by far the most secretive, with 62 per cent of the parents of children born after DI saying it was important to keep it a secret from others; 50 per cent expected to tell the children. In contrast, 96 per cent of all those in the survey who had or were still trying to have a child through IVF intended to tell the child. They generally *want* the children to know how special they are and how much trouble the parents went through to have them. Couples who hired surrogate mothers were a little less sure, but they generally planned to treat the subject openly. Logically, the child is least likely to need to know about an IVF conception where there was no donor involved, and yet this is the situation in which parents are most likely to plan to tell.

The key difference between DI and other methods is that the former usually involves male infertility and that other methods usually treat female infertility. AIH, artificial insemination using the husband's sperm, which can be used for either partner's problem, is more likely to be kept secret when used for male than for female infertility (Lasker and Borg 1989). It appears that the couples, and society as a whole, consider male infertility a much more serious stigma than female infertility; hence, secrecy is more for the protection of the infertile man (as well as for the physician and donor) than for the benefit of the child. It is much easier to keep DI secret than other forms of conception, and certainly easier than adoption. There is no legal transaction, and the mother has an apparently normal pregnancy and birth. The father's name is on the birth certificate, and often the attending obstetrician or midwife is unaware of the origin of the pregnancy. In addition, particularly in the United States, most physicians who offer DI and therapists who counsel prospective parents about donor insemination strongly advise the couples to maintain secrecy, never to tell the child or anyone else (Waltzer 1982).

The difference between men and women in feelings about secrecy can be a particularly difficult source of trouble. This difference is especially hard on a woman who needs to talk but feels she must comply with her husband's wishes to keep their infertility problems a secret. In our research (Lasker and Borg 1994), most couples said they agree with each other about whether or not to tell others of their experiences. Some couples, however, found this to be a problem. Generally, the men were more likely to want to keep everything secret (Lasker and Borg 1989; Back and Snowden 1988). A woman whose baby was conceived through donor insemination (also called AID) explained:

My husband insisted we tell no one about the AID procedure, and that was very hard for me. I felt that, in trying AID, I would be carrying another man's sperm, and if the process worked, I would be living with a 'lie' the rest of my life. I finally broke down and told a close friend. It felt like I was releasing an enormous pressure from my mind.

More parents are beginning to have a more open view of donor insemination. Our study showed that somewhat more people intended to tell their child about their origins than did not. Many were still uncertain, hoping to find an answer as the child grew older. The sample, like many in such studies, is not representative, since most of the people are members of the RESOLVE support organization. They are people who are willing to talk about infertility (Lasker and Borg 1994). But they are likely to represent a growing trend toward more openness about infertility. In Nielsen's study of Danish and Swedish couples at a Danish clinic, 51 per cent said they would tell the child when he or she grew up (Nielsen et al. 1995).

Most couples feel very torn between a desire to keep the information private and a strong need to talk to others about it. They are fearful of others' reactions. Yet they also talk about the stress of 'living a lie' and the wish to share such an important event with those to whom they are close. Schilling

(1995) reports that ten of thirty-four German couples interviewed five years after beginning insemination reported feeling 'oppressed by secrecy'.

Some people who use DI wish they could meet other people who have also used donor insemination so they could compare their feelings and experiences with each other. There are very few opportunities for this to happen, although a support group (DI Network) was established in 1993 in Great Britain, and RESOLVE in the United States provides an opportunity for people to contact each other (and more recently similar groups have now been established in Canada, Australia and New Zealand).

No matter how strongly they express a commitment to secrecy, most people included in studies of secrecy with DI had told at least one or two others. They are selective, often telling one set of parents but not the other, or certain friends they assumed would be sympathetic. But they have found it very difficult not to tell anyone at all. Klock and colleagues found that 38 per cent of the American couples they interviewed before insemination planned to tell someone else about DI, but only 27 per cent planned to tell the child (1994). As one father said, 'I couldn't tell him. You know, I will have raised him all his life and I just wouldn't have the heart to tell him. I'm afraid he'd be ashamed of me. It might break my heart as well as his.' Some experts claim that it is essential that children know their medical history and not assume they may share any medical problems experienced by the fathers who raise them. Some also fear that maintaining a secret about the child's origin is ultimately unhealthy for the family. Clamar emphasises this possibility: 'By its very nature, a secret is a potent force, assuming undue proportion and power within the family – an existential fact that remains unspoken, yet controls and colors the lives of the people involved' (1980: 176). Baran and Pannor, who began their study of donor insemination with a belief in the value of secrecy, were led by their findings to the opposite conclusion. They found that secrecy is 'lethal and destructive to the families involved. We are convinced that in all DI families, the need to maintain secrecy and anonymity has had an adverse effect upon all of the members' (1989: 13,152). Daniels and Taylor (1993) argue for the child's right to know his or her origins. The British Warnock Committee came out in favour of telling children about their conception (a position not held by most physicians) but still recommended that the donor be totally anonymous (Haimes 1993).

The decision to tell a child when he or she may never be able to find the donor creates an added dilemma for the parents, as noted earlier. The physicians who provide donor insemination usually counsel silence; social scientists who have studied DI almost always encourage openness. Yet most parents are opting for silence, and in some cases they are found to regret having decided to tell others (Nielsen *et al.* 1995; Klock *et al.* 1994).

Single heterosexual and lesbian women. For lesbians and heterosexual single women, the question of secrecy is totally different. The majority of single heterosexual and lesbian women who use DI do not keep the information secret (Golombok and Tasker 1994). They would rather that others, and the child, realise that the conception was planned and wanted, not the accidental result of a casual affair. Secrecy, then, is usually not a problem, nor is the issue of genetic inequality between parents. In Leiblum *et al.*'s (1995) study of single heterosexual and lesbian women who underwent DI, all of them planned to tell a child conceived through DI, and 57 per cent reported that they would like their prospective child to be able to meet the donor.

Conclusion

For those who do succeed, donor insemination, like many of the new technologies, is regarded very positively. Most studies indicate that parents of children conceived with DI are delighted with the results, and many of them return for another child. Yet the process also creates dilemmas for individual families to resolve. DI is certain to become increasingly common and more successful and therefore probably more public. Even so, it is likely to remain a secretive process, one producing great joy for many families but also many questions.

Many issues remain to be more carefully researched and considered; for example, the effects of DI on relationships, both heterosexual and homosexual. While there is very little known about how married couples cope with DI, there is essentially no research on the experience of lesbian couples. Is the partner who is not inseminated experiencing anxiety or jealousy? Should counselling be required for anyone who is having DI and for their partners? Should people who appear to be troubled by the process be excluded, or is this discriminatory?

We also know very little about the dynamics of decision-making within couples. Baran and Pannor (1989) suggest that often DI is actively promoted by physicians in almost the same breath with which they announce the man's infertility. Would it indeed be better to delay any discussion of DI until the man and his partner have had an opportunity to accept his infertility first? What are the consequences for couples, and for children, if the partners are ambivalent about going through with DI, or if one partner is more motivated than the other?

Since almost all studies of donor insemination are based on volunteers who select themselves, it is likely that there are many people who use DI who are simply not represented in research. It is also the case that programmes run by physicians and fertility centres attract a clientele almost all of whom can afford the treatment. Thus what little we do know is skewed towards white and relatively affluent people, mostly in the United States, Western Europe, and Oceania. A study from Cameroon suggests that there are very different issues of cultural norms and attitudes toward DI in that country than in countries where most studies are carried out (Savage 1992). How do social class, nationality, race, and ethnicity affect the likelihood of considering DI and the experience of using it? Are poorer women more likely to seek out their own donors, and if so, with what consequences? Baran and Pannor (1989) point out that the only working-class people in their study were lesbians who had found their own donors. In the study by Klock *et al.* (1994) of all couples seeking DI at a university-based infertility clinic, over three-quarters had a yearly income of at least US $50,000.

There is also very little known about how people select their own donors and the types of relationships which they have with the donor. What is the impact, for example, of having a brother of an infertile man donate sperm with which to inseminate his wife? There is the advantage that the child will share some genes with his or her father, but what happens to the family constellation in this kind of situation? Despite the court cases which reflect those situations in which there is conflict, there are many recipients of donor insemination who maintain very positive relationships with the donor, who may be known to the child and be an active and positive part of his or her life.

These are just a few of the questions which remain, the answering of which will help open the door on this practice, which has been in use for a long time but is still veiled in secrecy.

REFERENCES

Alexandre, Claude (1980) 'Difficulties encountered by infertile couples facing AID'. In G. David and W. Price, eds., *Human artificial insemination and semen preservation*. New York: Plenum Press.

Andrew, Lori (1985) *New conceptions: a consumer's guide to the newest infertility treatments*. New York: Ballantine.

Andrews, Frank M., Abbey, Antonia, and Halman, L. Jill (1991) 'Stress from infertility: marriage factors and subjective well-being of wives and husbands'. *Journal of Health and Social Behavior* 32: 238–53.

Anonymous (1985) 'AID doubts and feelings'. *RESOLVE Newsletter*, December, p. 2.

Araneta, M. R., Mascola, L., Eller, A., O'Neil, L., Ginsberg, M. M., Bursaw, M., Marik, J., Friedman, S., Sims, C. A., Rekart, M. L. *et al.* (1995) 'HIV transmission through donor artificial insemination'. *Journal of the American Medical Association* 273(11): 854–8.

Back, Kurt W. and Snowden, Robert (1988) 'The anonymity of the gamete donor'. *Journal of Psychosomatic Obstetrics and Gynecology* 9: 191–8.

Bailey, David (1995) 'Two lesbian couples appeal judge's denial of their adoption petitions'. *Chicago Daily Law Bulletin*, January 6: 1.

Baran, Annette and Pannor, Reuben (1989) *Lethal secrets: the shocking consequences and unsolved problems of artificial insemination*. New York: Warner Books.

Barlet, E. M. and Penney, L. L. (1994) 'Therapeutic donor insemination: fresh vs. frozen'. *Missouri Medicine* 91: 85–8.

Ben-Chetrit, A., Senoz, S., Greenblatt, E. M., and Casper, R. F. (1995) '*In vitro* fertilization outcome in the presence of severe male factor infertility'. *Fertility and Sterility* 63: 1,032–7.

Berger, David (1980) 'Couples' reaction to male infertility and donor insemination'. *American Journal of Psychiatry* 137: 1,047–9.

Bielawska-Batorowicz, Eleonora (1994) 'Artificial insemination by donor: an investigation of recipient couples' viewpoints'. *Journal of Reproductive and Infant Psychology* 12: 123–6.

Blaser, A., Maloigne-Katz, B., and Gigon, U. (1988) 'Effect of artificial insemination with donor semen on the psyche of the husband'. *Psychother. Psychosom.* 49: 17–21.

Bleckman, Elaine (1982) 'Are children with one parent at psychological risk? A methodological review'. *Journal of Marriage and the Family* 44: 179–95.

Brand, H. J. (1989) 'The influence of sex differences on the acceptance of infertility'. *Journal of Reproductive and Infant Psychology* 7: 127–31.

Brewaeys, A., Ponjaert-Kristoffersen, I., Van Steirteghem, A. C. and Devroey, P. (1993) 'Children from anonymous donors: an inquiry into homosexual and heterosexual parents' attitudes'. *Journal Psycho-som. Obstet. Gynaecol.* 14 Suppl.: 23–35.

Caplan, Arthur (1995) 'Needed: rules about corpses' sperm'. *The Houston Chronicle*, 4 February, p. 2

Clamar, Aphrodite (1980) 'Psychological implications of donor insemination'. *American Journal of Psychoanalysis* 40: 173–77.

Cornacchia, Cheryl (1994) 'Lesbians face discrimination in Canada, lawyer charges'. *The Gazette* (Montreal). 18 July, C3.

Danesh-Meyer, H. V., Gillett W. R., and Daniels, K. R. (1993) 'Withdrawal from a donor insemination program'. *Australian New Zealand Journal of Obstetrics and Gynaecology* 33: 187–90.

Daniels, Ken R. (1994) 'Adoption and donor insemination: factors influencing couples' choices'. *Child Welfare* 73: 5–14.

Daniels, K. R. and Taylor, K. (1993) 'Secrecy and openness in donor insemination'. *Politics and the Life Sciences* 12.

Dean, Malcolm (1994) 'The right to be a family: British lesbian couple have made raising children their priority'. *The Gazette* (Montreal), 18 July, C3.

d'Elicio, Giuseppe, Campana, Aldo, and Mornaghini, L. (1980) 'Psychodynamic discussions with couples requesting AID', in G. David and W. Price, eds., *Human artificial insemination and semen preservation*. New York: Plenum Press.

Draye, Mary Ann, Woods, Nancy Fugate, and Mitchell, Ellen (1988) 'Coping with infertility in couples: gender differences'. *Health Care for Women International* 9: 163–75.

Dreyfous, Leslie (1991) 'Gay couples are redefining parenthood'. *The Morning Call* (Allentown, PA), 21 April, p. A4.

Englert, Y. (1994) 'Artificial insemination of single women and lesbian women with donor semen'. *Human Reproduction* 9: 1,969–71.

Flaks, David K., Ficher, Ilda, Masterpasqua, Frank, and Joseph, Gregory (1995) 'Lesbians choosing motherhood: a comparative study of lesbian and heterosexual parents and their children'. *Developmental Psychology* 31: 105–14.

Golombok, Susan and Tasker, Fiona (1994) 'Donor insemination for single heterosexual and lesbian women: issues concerning the welfare of the child'. *Human Reproduction*, 9: 1,972–6.

Greil, Arthur L. (1991) *Not yet pregnant: infertile couples in contemporary America.* New Brunswick: Rutgers University Press.

Greil, Arthur L., Leitko, Thomas, and Porter, Karen L. (1988) 'Infertility: his and hers'. *Gender and Society*, 2: 172–99.

Greil, Arthur L., Porter, Karen L., and Leitke, Thomas A. (1989) 'Sex and intimacy among infertile couples'. *Journal of Psychology and Human Sexuality* 2: 117–38.

Haimes, Erica (1993) 'Issues of gender in gamete donation'. *Social Science and Medicine* 36: 85–93.

Hartman, Lili (1985) 'Thoughts from the fertile partner', *RESOLVE Newsletter*, September.

Henry, V. L. (1993) 'A tale of three women: a survey of the rights and responsibilities of unmarried women who conceive by alternative insemination and a model for legislative reform'. *American Journal Law and Medicine* 19: 285–311.

Holding, Reynolds (1994) 'Sperm donor is legal dad, court rules'. *The San Francisco Chronicle*, 19 November, B12.

Humphrey, M. and Humphrey, H. (1987) 'Marital relationships in couples seeking donor insemination'. *Journal of Biosocial Science* 19: 209–19.

(1993) 'Vasectomy as a reason for donor insemination'. *Social Science and Medicine* 37: 363–6.

Klock, Susan C., Jacob, Mary Casey and Maier, Donald (1994) 'A prospective study of donor insemination recipients: secrecy, privacy, and disclosure'. *Fertility and Sterility* 62: 477–84.

Lasker, Judith and Borg, Susan (1989) 'Secrecy and the new reproductive technologies'. In Linda Whiteford and Marilyn Poland, eds., *New approaches to human reproduction; social and ethical dimensions.* Boulder: Westview Press.

(1994) *In search of parenthood; coping with infertility and high-tech conception.* Philadelphia: Temple University Press.

Ledward, R. S., Symonds, E. M., and Eynon, S. (1982) 'Social and environmental factors as criteria for success in artificial insemination by donor'. *Journal of Biosocial Science* 14: 263–75.

Leiblum, S. R., Palmer, M. G., and Spector, I. P. (1995) 'Non-traditional mothers: single heterosexual/lesbian women and lesbian couples electing motherhood via donor insemination'. *Journal of Psychosomatic Obstet. Gynaecol.* 16: 11–20.

Levie, L. H. (1967) 'An inquiry into the psychological effects on parents of artificial insemination with donor sperm'. *Eugenics Review*, 59, 97–105.

McCann, Sheila R. (1994) 'Judge gives lesbian right to visitation with ex-partner's child'. *Salt Lake Tribune*, 20 November, B1.

McGuire, Maureen and Alexander, Nancy (1985) 'Artificial insemination of single women'. *Fertility and Sterility* 43: 182–4.

McNamee, Tom (1994). 'Lesbian, gay parents increasing, but hard to count'. *Chicago Sun-Times*, 28 November, 4.

Mason, Mary Claire (1993) *Male infertility: men talking*. London: Routledge.

Milsom, Ian and Bergman, Per (1982) 'A study of parental attitudes after donor insemination'. *Acta Obstetrica et Gynecologica Scandinavica*, 61, 125–8.

Nachtigall, R. D. (1994) 'Donor insemination and human immunodeficiency virus: a risk/benefit analysis'. *American Journal of Obstetrics and Gynecology* 170: 1,692–6.

Nielsen, Anders Faurskov, Pedersen, Bjorn, and Lauritsen, Jorgen G. (1995) 'Psychosocial aspects of donor insemination: attitudes and opinions of Danish and Swedish donor insemination patients to psychosocial information being supplied to offspring and relatives'. *Acta Obstetrica et Gynecologica Scandinavica* 74: 45–50.

Office of Technology Assessment, US Congress (1988) *Artificial insemination: practice in the US: summary of a 1987 survey.* Washington, DC: US Government Printing Office.

Orenstein, Peggy (1995) 'Looking for a donor to call Dad'. *The New York Times Sunday Magazine*, 18 June, 28.

Ostrom, Carol M. and King, Warren (1993). 'Infertility clinic accused of past bias: women say lesbians, singles turned away by UW facility'. *The Seattle Times*, 21 November.

Owens, D. J., Edelmann, R. E., and Humphrey, M. E. (1993) 'Male infertility and donor insemination: couples' decisions, reactions, and counselling needs'. *Human Reproduction* 8: 880–5.

Palermo, G. D., Cohen, J., Alikani, M., Adler, A., and Rosenwaks, Z. (1995) 'Intracytoplasmic sperm injection: a novel treatment for all forms of male factor infertility'. *Fertility and Sterility* 63: 1,231–40.

Pies, Cheri A. (1989) 'Lesbians and the choice to parent'. *Marriage and Family Review* 14: 137–54.

Prattke, T. W. and Gass-Sternas, K. A. (1993) 'Appraisal, coping, and emotional health of infertile couples undergoing donor insemination'. *Journal of Obstetrics and Gynecol. Neonatal Nursing* 22: 516–27.

Reading, Anthony E., Sledmere, Caroline M., and Cox, David N. (1982) 'A survey of patient attitudes toward artificial insemination by donor'. *Journal of Psychosomatic Research* 26: 429–33.

Rosenkvist, Hans (1981) 'Donor insemination: a prospective socio-psychiatric investigation of 48 couples'. *Danish Medical Bulletin* 28: 133–48.

Rubin, Bernard (1965) 'Psychological aspects of human artificial insemination'. *Archives of General Psychiatry* 13: 121–32.

Rubin, Sylvia (1995) 'Family secrets'. *The San Francisco Chronicle*, 15 January, p. 1.

Savage, Olayinka Margaret Njikam (1993) 'Artificial donor insemination in Yaounde: some socio-cultural considerations'. *Social Science and Medicine* 35: 907–13.

Schilling, G. (1995) 'Family secrets exemplified by heterologous insemination'. *Psychother. Psychosom. Med. Psychol.* 45: 16–23 (English abstract).

Schover, Leslie R., Collins, Robert L., and Richards, Susan (1992) 'Psychological aspects of donor insemination: evaluation and follow-up of recipient couples'. *Fertility and Sterility* 57: 583–90.

Schover, L. R., Greenhalgh, L. F., Richards, S. I., and Collins, R. L. (1994) 'Psychological screening and the success of donor insemination'. *Human Reproduction* 9: 176–8.

Selby, Holly (1995) 'More gay couples becoming parents'. *The Palm Beach Post*, 15 January, 7D.

Shenfield, Francoise (1994) 'Particular requests in donor insemination: comments on the medical duty of care and the welfare of the child'. *Human Reproduction* 9: 1,976–7.

Simons, Marlise (1995) 'Uproar over twins, and a Dutch couple's anguish'. *The New York Times*, 28 June, A3.

Snowden, R., Mitchell, G. D., and Snowden, E. M. (1983) *Artificial reproduction: a social investigation*. London: George Allen and Unwin.

'Sperm banks and clinics, where to go' (1994) *Washingtonian Magazine*, March.

Stephenson, Patricia St Clair and Wagner G. Marsden (1991) 'Turkey-baster babies; a view from Europe'. *The Milbank Quarterly* 69: 45–50.

Stephenson, Patricia (1993) 'Ovulation induction during treatment of infertility: an assessment of the risks'. In Patricia Stephenson and Marsden G. Wagner, eds., *Tough choices: in vitro fertilization and the reproductive technologies*. Philadelphia: Temple University Press, pp. 97–121.

Stone, Sergio (1980) 'Complications and pitfalls of artificial insemination'. *Clinical Obstetrics and Gynecology* 23: 667–82.

Strong, Carson and Schinfeld, Jay (1984) 'The single woman and artificial insemination by donor'. *Journal of Reproductive Medicine* 29: 293–9.

Tucker, M. J. (1995) 'Micromanipulative and conventional insemination strategies for assisted reproductive technology'. *American Journal of Obstetrics Gynecology* 172 (part 2): 773–8.

Utian, Wulf, Goldfarb, James, and Rosenthal, Miriam (1983) 'Psychological aspects of infertility'. In L. Dennerstein and G. D. Burrows, eds., *Handbook of psychosomatic obstetrics and gynecology*. New York: Elsevier.

Waltzer, Herbert (1982) 'Psychological and legal aspects of artificial insemination (AID): an overview'. *American Journal of Psychotherapy* 36: 91–102.

Zoldbrod, Aline (1988) 'The emotional distress of the artificial insemination patient'. *Medical Psychotherapy* 1: 161–72.

3   Families created through donor insemination

Robert and Elizabeth Snowden

Introduction

Most people would accept the proposition that sexual relationships, the birth of children and the nurture of infants and young children are normally contained within the set of relationships we call the family. In many respects the family is an elusive concept which describes relationships with which we are all familiar but which, on closer examination, we find difficult to define with precision. Because of our close personal experience of family life we are apt to assume we know what we mean when we speak of the 'family'. Moreover, it is usual to assume that the word has the same meaning for us that it has for others and that our experience is similar to that of other people. However, while the recognition that family members have a special relationship with each other appears to be ubiquitous, the form and quality of these relationships vary between and within societies and even in the same family group over time.

What makes the study of these relationships even more difficult is that the thoughts one brings to bear on such a study have largely been structured by the very relationships being studied. The subjective nature of family relationships is one which is not readily amenable to objective assessment or measurement using the traditional tools of science and for this reason their detailed study remains either neglected or problematic.

In our personal lives most of us are exposed to the importance of subjective experiences; indeed, it is these positive or negative feelings which tend to hold most meaning for us. While attempts have been made to scale or measure such subjective feelings, these attempts have generally not succeeded beyond what most researchers would regard as a superficial level. However, this inability to assess the impact of subjective experiences in a way which permits objective measurement should not be allowed to diminish the significance of these experiences or lead to an underestimation of their value.

While the special group of people described as family members exerts deep and significant subjective influences of a very pervasive kind, the

33

concept of the family also describes an institution which socialises individuals to become members of a particular society through the inculcation of society-specific values which maintain that society both in the present and from one generation to the next. The birth of children and their socialisation as members of a given society has been, and continues to be, an underlying concern in all societies. The rules and norms by which reproduction and socialisation take place may vary between societies and in the same society over time but they are pervasive and more powerful than we often recognise.

Of all family relationships, the most important are those which, in one way or another, affect and are affected by the birth process. As Davis (1984) has noted, 'all marital and familial phenomena ultimately come back to connections through birth'. The birth of a child has implications not just for the child's parents but also for a much wider and larger group of surrounding individuals.

Family relationships are normally based on biological links and possess varying degrees of closeness to the individual. Radcliffe-Brown (1950) has identified seven primary relatives (mother, father, daughter, son, sister, brother, spouse), with secondary relatives (primary relatives of one's primary relatives) and tertiary relatives (primary relatives of one's secondary relatives) occupying a widening circle of family members. Parents, children and siblings usually take these biological links for granted; indeed, to question such links too closely is likely to be considered improper. Whilst most relatives share a common biological inheritance, the link between spouses is of a different kind. At first encounter, spouses do not share a known predisposing biological link but one that is usually presumed as a likely consequence of their union. In other words there is an expectation that their genes will be combined in the future through the conception and birth of their own progeny. This is not to say this event inevitably takes place but for most people, the expectation is one which bears considerable influence. This biologically based distribution of relatives contains a clear hierarchy of family members attracting different levels of commitment to each other.

When considered from this perspective, donor insemination represents an absent biological link in those families where this method of procreation is used. A couple bringing up a child conceived by donor insemination cannot look at their offspring and see a mingling of their genes; their union has not resulted in the procreation of 'their own' progeny. For them, such a child, though much loved, is qualitatively different from a child who is biologically linked to them both and who, in turn, retrospectively provides a biological link between them. This has implications for themselves, for the child, and also for their wider kinsfolk. If this were not so the secrecy surrounding the donor insemination procedure, the desire for donor anonymity and the public uncertainty leading to the need for regulation would not have arisen as it has in many societies. The conflicting claims and theoretical arguments about nature versus nurture, genetic versus environmental, and the biological versus the sociological interpretations of personal identity all hold particular significance for couples whose children represent a planned discontinuity between biological and social parenting through the use of DI.

Family relationships and DI: a research project

The means of alleviating childlessness caused by male infertility using DI have been available in the United Kingdom for just over half a century. In September 1940 a pioneering woman doctor, practising in the West of England, first began to provide DI to couples who were childless because of male infertility. She continued this provision for the next forty years and by 1980 a total of 899 couples had undergone donor insemination, and as a result 480 children had been born. This practitioner was unusually far-sighted in the provision of this service in that she appreciated the social significance of the treatment she was providing should a child be conceived and born. Her work remains unique in the United Kingdom in that she attempted to keep in regular contact with couples who had successfully used the service. Over a period of forty years she received, and stored, regular information from many of these couples about the development of their children and the well-being of the family which had been created through the use of DI. This led, at the end of the 1970s, to the development of a research programme to investigate the social and psychological implications of DI on family relationships, both within the nuclear family so created and between that family and wider kin. This research is still on-going (in 1995) and incorporates the collection of both retrospective and prospective information concerning the experiences and expectations of these family members (Snowden and Snowden 1994).

As a first step, a retrospective study of the experience of couples undergoing DI between 1940 and 1980 based on correspondence and records held at the treatment centre was undertaken. The correspondence contained letters describing the effect of DI on the relationship of this couple, the development of their child(ren) and the progress of their family life. This correspondence provided insights into the issues which were thought to be important by the couples concerned and helped to identify areas which could be explored further during interview. The second phase of the study took place during 1981 when all couples who had a baby between 1977 and 1980 following DI provided in this same practice were asked if they would be willing to be interviewed about their experience; fifty-seven couples with pre-school age children were interviewed. Some couples had remained in contact with the practitioner over several decades and their sons and daughters were now adult and no longer living in the parental home. The opportunity was taken to interview ten of these couples who had a lengthy experience of DI parenting. The third phase of the study took place in 1990 when twenty-nine of these same couples whose children had now reached secondary school age were interviewed a second time. Contact is being maintained with these couples, and it is hoped to conduct a third round of interviews when their children reach adulthood. (All unattributed quotations in this chapter are taken from this ongoing research.)

The reporting of this research has, to date, been confined to the study of family relationships from the perspective of the married couple seeking DI treatment as a means of resolving their childlessness. Discussions have also taken place with a small number of adults who are aware they were conceived by DI and with donors and DI service providers. Inevitably, the bulk of the information about relationships with the child within the family has been taken from the parents' perception of these relationships.

The parents' experience of DI

Following the first round of interviews with parents of pre-school age children it was noted:

The overall impression gained from the interviews was that the vast majority of couples was immensely grateful that their involuntary childless state had been resolved. Almost without exception they had no regrets about their decision to employ DI and with hindsight would make the same decision again. This did not mean, however, that they had discovered no hitches or problems. Many couples felt that some of their experiences, and the way they had dealt with certain situations, had not been ideal; given the opportunity, they would have wished to change things in certain respects. All the husbands (and wives) appeared to have accepted the children willingly and happily; indeed some of the fathers had a particularly close relationship with their children and appeared to be deeply involved in child care and family life. Because their children had been achieved after considerable heartache, and after much effort, they were particularly valued and loved and the couples tended to find parenting particularly rewarding and satisfying. (Snowden, Mitchell and Snowden 1983: 81)

In reporting on the second round of interviews undertaken eight years later it was stated:

Our overwhelming impression was that the great majority of these families were functioning well, and the children were valued, loved and enjoyed. This opinion was based not only on what the couples said, but on our observations of their interactions during a lengthy and informal interview and on our assessment of the ambience of their homes. The majority of the couples appeared more mature, affluent and self-confident than we remembered them eight years ago. The couples did have problems in their family life, but saw them as normal problems experienced in all families; they did not identify them as resulting from donor insemination. They were extremely grateful this technique had allowed them to become a family; without exception grandparents and other relatives had accepted the children. (Snowden and Snowden 1991: 8).

Two couples were known to have divorced since the initial interview and one mother had been widowed.

Despite the general impression of well-being among these families it should not be construed that DI parenting is a simple matter. Though the medical procedure itself is simple, the emotional, social and psychological implications of resolving childlessness this way are complex. Among couples there is a manifest desire to repress the experience of DI and most couples assert they never think about their children's donor conception. However, even as this statement is made, a second often follows which describes a general feeling that it is unsettling to think too deeply about how their children had been conceived. The majority of couples prefer not to acknowledge, even to each other, their recourse to DI.

During the planning of the second round of interviews and as parents found themselves once more being invited to think and talk about their experience of DI parenthood, most found the topic of discussion uncomfortable and some gave this as the reason for wishing not to take part in further discussion. It would seem these couples had not fully resolved their feelings about male infertility, the means they had chosen to solve their childlessness and the implications of this for their relationship with each other. It is as if the presence of a child created with the aid of a third party threatens family relationships in some way and the most obvious means of dealing with this uncertain situation is to avoid talking, or thinking, about it.

This situation is not helped when DI is presented as a straightforward medical treatment for male infertility. In almost all respects DI is neither a medical procedure nor a medical treatment in the generally accepted use of these terms. Because the condition of infertility is not treated, even indirectly, when DI is provided, the involvement of the medical profession may appear difficult to justify; the unfit husband receives no medical treatment whatsoever whilst his fit wife receives the full attention of the medical team. Some husbands were very conscious of their continuing infertility even when recourse to the medical profession and to DI had resulted in the birth of a son or daughter. Such men are liable to feel ignored or forgotten by the medical team. DI does not enable an infertile man to reproduce, to procreate, to sire a descendant, to experience a kind of genetic or temporal immortality as he recognises his own features in those of his offspring; put simply, DI may resolve childlessness but it does not cure infertility.

Biological and nurturing family relationships

The central complexity in any use of donor gametes to resolve childlessness is the resulting disjunction between the biological and nurturing relationships with the child so created. In the case of DI the child has two 'fathers'; the semen provider who acts as the genetic father and the mother's partner who provides nurturance as the child's 'social' father.

Male infertility is experienced as a life crisis. It could perhaps be argued that in terms of biological significance, an inability to reproduce has greater significance even than that of death. It is interesting to note that the psychological stages of the response to a diagnosis of terminal illness described by Kübler-Ross (1969) (starting with denial and ending with an eventual acceptance) are similar to those described by Eck-Menning (1977) in relation to a diagnosis of infertility. During one interview the father of two children conceived by DI said:

My major hang-up really was based on this rather metaphysical notion of genetic immortality. What depressed me most of all, and overwhelmed me mentally, was this idea that at this point my genetic channel stops. That's the end. And that was the most chilling thing I had to take on board. I must be frank and say that I still wish that I could father a child; this is still a faint note of sadness to me. But it doesn't intrude into my relationship with these two children, because I can really put my hand on my heart and say I wouldn't really change them. But I think if somebody suddenly discovered that my fertility had come back I would want to try most vigorously to have a child. But I think that's a very primeval and natural response.

DI does not enable a man to reproduce; it is a conservative social measure which allows for the creation of a family unit by permitting the man's wife or partner to conceive another man's baby without sexual contact. In other words, it allows the couple to maintain the physical, sexual integrity of their relationship whilst resolving their childlessness. This permits the apparent presence of the three major functions of family life (the integrity of sexual relationships, the bearing of children and their socialisation) but, in historical terms, in a novel way. What separates DI from other forms of family building (eg. adoption) is that the female partner conceives and bears a child using gametes provided by another, usually unknown, male. In other circumstances, such behaviour would provide strong justification for the dissolution of the relationship between the couple concerned resulting in the break-up of the group as a family unit. With this in mind, it should not come as a surprise to learn that recourse to DI in the early days was legally considered to be equivalent to adultery and was not to be encouraged.

During the interviews among family members it was noticeable that there was confusion about the meaning of fatherhood in terms of the genetic and nurturing functions of this role. It was common for the partners of the mothers of children conceived by DI to refer frequently to the semen provider as the 'real' father, but then to forcefully claim paternity for 'my' child. It was not so much that these men were able to acknowledge and feel comfortable with the distinction between genitor and pater (the denial of the personality or even the presence of a donor was also commonplace) but rather the expression of an incoherent feeling of uncertainty and unease resulting from an underlying sense of confusion concerning the relationship between himself and the child. The inevitable consequence of this confusion for fathers is that the children created in this way are also likely to experience a duality of interpretation when attempting to describe the feelings they experience in their perceived relationships with their father(s).

In all societies there have always been socially approved procedures by which the role of a parent can be defined legally. While the genetic link provides *a priori* evidence for such legal rights, special arrangements are present for dealing with applications for adoption where the presumed genetic link is absent. Similarly, many societies have laws which define the conditions in which the role of parent can be removed or denied. There is a ubiquitous interest in the creation and dissolution by the state of the social unit described as the family. Who is and who is not defined as the mother or father of a child has far-reaching implications for individuals both in the present (which is informed by the past) and in the future. Personal identity based on perceived ancestry, combined with temporal immortality based on the creation of descendants, known and yet to be born, is a powerful mix contributing to what Lindahl and Back (1987) describes as lineage consciousness. As is often the case, it is those who are not in a position to take such matters for granted who provide the greatest insights into what is taken as the norm. So it is for the sterile male who, in terms of his genetic links, demonstrates in the same person a discontinuity between genetic and social paternity while being the intentional creator of a child with a partner who demonstrates no such discontinuity.

In order to deal with the social uncertainty engendered by the introduction of gamete donation, some countries have introduced laws for the control of what is generally described as the 'new reproductive technologies'. Among the most comprehensive legislation is that contained in the Human Fertilisation and Embryology Act (1990) of the United Kingdom. This law bestows legal paternity on the male partner of the woman conceiving by DI; the semen provider has no rights or duties, either in the present or the future, in relation to the paternity of the child. This law recognises the infertile male partner's role in agreeing to the creation of the child (rather than providing the necessary gametes) and to taking responsibility for the child's welfare. In this way, DI parents may be identified as the 'social' creators of the child, the birth of whom would not occur but for the decision made from within that couple's relationship (Snowden and Snowden 1993). Hill (1991) uses a similar justification for the recognition of these parents but prefers to describe such couples as 'intentional' parents. He argues that owing to the element of planning and prior agreement by the couple, 'intentional' parents have a respectable claim to being procreators and goes on to assert that their legal right to parenthood should even take precedence over the claims of biological parents because of the planned intention of their agreed behaviour and the acceptance of responsibility for its results. Children born following DI are among the most planned and carefully created of any being born, and the skill and thought involved in the creation of families by this procedure should be recognised.

It is noteworthy that in the case of DI, the maternal role is not questioned. The assumption remains absolute that the genetic link together with the bearing of the child is sufficient to determine motherhood. There is some evidence that in Western cultures, the biological tie with the mother is seen as more significant than that with the father. Edwards (1993) found that step-siblings who have the same mother but different fathers are perceived as being closer than those who have the same father but different mothers. It is widely recognised in legal terms that a child's biological relationship to its putative father is, in general, less certain than that of the biological tie with the mother who gave birth. Hill states that in law 'in general fatherhood is a status which is predominantly a function of the family relationship. More specifically, it is a status accorded to men who entertain certain kinds of relationship with the mother and the child. Ultimately, there is only a contingent relationship between this relational status and the genetic connection between putative father and child' (1991: 372). O'Brien (1981) suggests that men, who are less close to their children than are mothers because of the birth tie, nevertheless have a need to identify their children in a meaningful way, and do this by naming all children born into their family as theirs.

It is the combination of the maternal genetic link and the act of child bearing that creates the close bond between mother and child. Despite legal recognition for the birth mother, it is probable that in the minds of most observers, the genetic link is assumed to be the most powerful in terms of social (and therefore personal) recognition and identity. It is this continuing assumption that places the role of the gamete provider in an uncertain position concerning paternity. While legislation may prescribe, and proscribe, who is to be legally regarded as 'the father' to the satisfaction of lawyers and legislators, it is less certain that this legal definition of father-hood removes the uncertainty surrounding the psychological needs of the family members in terms of the perceived relationships they have with each other which have such a powerful influence on self identity.

Some of the importance which attaches to biological ties of family members is because of their unalterable nature. These ties may not be permanent in the sense that they can be legally revoked; yet despite this legal revocability the biological tie remains, unchangeable and constant, and cannot be undone. This unchangeable nature of the biological tie is absent in DI fathering. Though DI fathers are 'intentional' fathers (as described by Hill 1991) at the outset of the DI procedure, it is possible they could come to regret that 'intention' at some later date and so distance themselves from the child who was created partly as a result of their agree-ment and the personal support of the mother. In the absence of a biolog-ical imperative through a genetic link, the possibility of a subsequent denial of responsibility for the child is keenly felt by some mothers and even by some of the DI fathers. Most of the 'intentional' fathers interviewed in the study were aware of this potential difficulty in family relationships: to love and accept a baby or young child as one's own is one thing; to maintain that acceptance throughout childhood, and particularly during the (antici-pated) period of adolescence, is another. One married male partner said:

I suppose its the point of concern that adoptive parents have, that when you get to adolescence and the balloon goes up as it were, its easy to shelve off responsibility by perhaps even in anger actually saying 'Well he isn't mine anyway. This is nothing to do with me.' And it does worry me that one hopes one is going to have the equanimity and stability to weather any storms of that kind. (Snowden and Snowden 1993: 131).

Researchers in the field of adoption studies generally place less empha-sis on the genetic link between parents and children, preferring to accord prime importance to the nurturance of family relationships. However, there is generally acknowledgement of the adopted child's need for knowledge of his/her biological ties. Triseliotis found that in the development of a secure personal identity, the paramount factor was the quality of the child's rela-tionship with adoptive parents. In most cases where adoptees arranged meetings with biological parents, Triseliotis found that 'blood brought the two sides together, but it could not create relationships for them' (1993: 196). McWhinnie (1993) also stresses that nurturing parents are usually seen by children as their 'real' parents. She believes this offers a more per-suasive argument to encourage parents to be open with their children than to make an appeal to children's 'right' to know that they have been adopted. The relative importance attached to the natural or nurturing links between parents and children in the creation of family relationships tends to be determined by the circumstances surrounding the particular situation. But clearly, both are important.

Whilst recognising that the basis and fabric of family life is concerned with perceived biological links and nurturing relationships, it appears futile to attempt to separate them or even to attempt a realistic measure of their relative importance. As Haimes (1993) reminds us, comparative studies from both history and anthropology have shown that the family derives its authority and status partly from an appeal to the natural basis of the biological relationship between the generations. Nevertheless biological links are always defined and understood within a specific cultural context. McNeil (1990) goes further when approaching this topic from the social rather than the biological end of the continuum by arguing that there are no 'biological givens' easily separable from the social realm.

In terms of the families where the biological and social ties have been deliberately separated for one of the adult members but not for the other through recourse to DI, discussions with couples would suggest that DI parents tend to emphasise the biological or the nurturing links depending on which of these alternative views allows their relationship and sense of connectedness with their children to be maximised. For example, when couples explain their preference for DI over adoption they tend to emphasise the importance of biological links with the child. One mother said: 'With adoption, you don't always know much about the parents. With DI you know it is half mine, and you know all the donors are carefully vetted.' Later in the interview the same mother commented:

some adopted children are from teenage mothers, perhaps with not very good backgrounds, and you don't know how that child might turn out. Because I know a lot of it depends on environment, but it is partly heredity, and I think in a way you can feel more sure with DI than with adoption that you are likely to end up with a reasonable outcome.

Another mother recalled her experience before her own child, conceived by DI, was born:

I looked after a friend's baby for a week once, and it was about a year old then and it kept doing things, and I kept thinking 'I wonder if my baby would have done that at that age?' And I thought if I adopt a baby I'm going to spend the rest of my life thinking that – saying I wonder if my baby would have done that.

However, when referring to the relationship between the child and the mother's partner, emphasis was repeatedly given to the role of nurturance by the couples interviewed. Comments such as 'Apart from not putting the sperm there [my husband] has been there the whole time' were made frequently. Also common was the idea that the male partner was the child's father 'to all intents and purposes'. One husband said: 'I feel very strongly that we do impart more than the major part of the child, rather than it being hereditary factors. I believe the parents create the child, rather than the child creating itself.'

However, while emphasising the biological link between the child and the mother and the nurturing link with the mother's partner, couples generally tended to discount the biological link between the child and the semen provider. One husband said: 'As far as we were concerned the baby would be 99 per cent [my wife's] and 1 per cent lent from someone'. His wife developed this idea: 'That's always been your [her husband's] view, hasn't it? Which in a sense is true enough. After all, the woman carries it for nine months so it's got to be more of the woman, hasn't it, if you look at it that way?' Another mother said: 'While I was pregnant it never entered my head – or I never really thought that it wasn't [my husband's] child, because it's [the DI procedure] so impersonal.' Another mother explained: 'I know it sounds silly but [my son] is like a clone of me.'

It had been hypothesised that couples would prefer second and subsequent DI children to be conceived from the same semen provider as the first child. This would minimise the number of extraneous biological links within the family being created. However, among the interview sample in the study being reported there was much less concern about this than had been anticipated; one explanation for this appears to be the discounting of the relevance and role of the semen provider by the DI parents. However, among parents who admit to a close, but clinical, interest in the selection of the semen donor and who state an intention to be more open with their children about their DI origins, different attitudes hold. Mays (1994), who is the mother of two children conceived by DI, and a founder member of *DI Network*, a self-help support group for DI parents, states that her greatest source of anxiety when her second child was planned was the knowledge that this conception would be the product of a different semen provider. Because of their need for DI, she and her husband had of necessity to accept a third dimension in their relationship and they did not want to contemplate a fourth. In addition she believes that where donated gametes are used, and regardless of the relationship siblings ultimately develop, there may be psychological benefits from the knowledge that one's brother or sister is a full sibling. The tension between the perceived importance of biological and nurturing ties was further illustrated in those families where there were naturally conceived as well as donor conceived children; some fathers were conscious they may be tempted to prefer their biologically related children over those with whom they exercised a similar nurturing role but in the absence of a biological link. The mothers of adopted and donor conceived children had a similar fear they might demonstrate or feel a preference for their biological children. One of the mothers had delivered her donor conceived child by caesarean section; she used this fact to reduce the importance of the birth link, and asserted that she felt the same about both children because 'both my children were handed to me'. The importance of genetic links had also been perceived by a child whose mother had divorced and remarried. His stepfather had two children from a previous marriage and they visited alternate weekends. His mother said: 'I think its sometimes hard for [my son] to see him with them, its difficult – there is a difference.'

Two parents who were themselves adopted also give a further illustration of the perceived importance of biological links to the individuals concerned. One, a woman, preferred DI as a means of solving her childlessness because she felt a need for a biological link which would give her a sense of reproductive continuity: 'I wanted a baby of my own, because not having a mother of my own I wanted a baby of my own.' The other adopted parent, an infertile husband, had recently tried to seek information about his birth mother:

As I grew older I began to think more about my situation. I felt isolated. There was nobody behind me and nobody in front. I know I am the father of the boys, make no mistake about that, but there isn't that link. There was just me on my own. Because I was adopted I didn't have a link going backward, and because I just happen to be infertile as well I don't have anyone coming on forward from me. I haven't come from anywhere and I'm not going on anywhere.

And yet this man's situation also amply illustrates the importance and strength of nurturing links; he has a very good and close relationship with his adoptive mother who lives close by. He went on to say: 'I knew I had to find out about my story before I would be satisfied and rest content. But it doesn't make any difference to how I feel about her, she is my mother, she always will be.' His sons also have a very warm and affectionate relationship with their grandmother. We saw this for ourselves when she arrived at the end of the interview; the mutual love and affection was plain to see. And yet biological links are doubly absent in this relationship: absent between the grandmother and the boys' father, and absent between the father and his sons. The grandmother is aware that the boys are conceived by DI, and the boys are aware that their father is adopted, yet these relationships remain strong and valued. However, despite his own experience and this evidence of a strong and enduring nurturing relationship with his almost teenage sons, this father is adamant that he will not inform them of their different biological origins and states he has no intention of providing them with this information in the future.

It seems that to the uncertainty surrounding the discontinuity between genetic and social parenting must be added the confusion created by the holding of sometimes opposing points of view depending on which family member is being considered; mother, father, gamete donor, half-siblings by different donors and by the presence of naturally conceived siblings. Add to this the complicating experiences of adoption, divorce, re-marriage and step-parenting and it is not surprising to find that most couples deal with the special situation in which they find themselves by adopting a stance of secrecy.

Family membership and the sharing of information about DI

Biological ties may be prospective as well as retrospective. A couple will be biologically unrelated until they produce a child. This child will then possess a shared genetic inheritance from that couple and so form a prospective biological tie linking that couple together. In this way, children are often seen as cementing a relationship. Likewise grandparents normally share a prospective biological link with a daughter-in-law or son-in-law after the birth of a grandchild. Because this intermingling of genes is missing when children are conceived by DI, many parents resorting to this form of family creation take refuge in maintaining a stance of secrecy (especially from those family members closest to them) about their recourse to DI. The question for couples concerning whether to share, or to withhold information about recourse to DI is clearly one which does not have an easy answer. Holmes has argued that there is no resolution to this question by stating in reference to family relationships that 'openness devastates; secrecy undermines'(1993: 181). Holmes, while claiming DI is not a satisfactory solution to male infertility, goes on to state that couples should not be presented with a solution to their childlessness which introduces an ethical situation which has no satisfactory solution. Lauritzen (1993) would agree that there are ethical difficulties inherent in DI; yet he pursues a more positive and optimistic approach, arguing that families can satisfactorily be created in this way provided couples work together towards a mutually agreed rationale for accepting DI treatment which maintains the integrity of the process of procreation, the integrity of their relationship, and that of their relationships with other kin. In our present culture, which expects technology to be able to solve most problems, it is not realistic to expect couples to decline DI as a solution to their problem because of inherent ethical difficulties. Lauritzen's approach in attempting to define conditions under which DI can be undertaken with integrity and without deception would appear to be a more constructive course of action.

When the family members studied in this research project conceived their children it was taken for granted *by those providing the service* that keeping

DI secret was the only sensible approach; the woman would become pregnant, apparently in the normal way, and 'no-one need ever know' about recourse to DI. Thirty-three of the fifty-seven couples with young children who were initially interviewed, claimed they had informed no one outside the medical profession about their DI treatment. Only two couples stated they made this information generally available among family members and had also allowed friends and neighbours to become aware. When couples were re-interviewed eight years later, their decision about whether or not to maintain a stance of secrecy had remained constant; no couple had changed their mind since the previous interview.

Since the inquiry into the new reproductive technologies contained in the Warnock Report (1984), and the Human Fertilisation and Embryology Act, 1990 which resulted from this report, the assumption that a stance of secrecy about DI is appropriate has been called into question. Official pronouncements now advise that couples should consider the value of informing the child about the means of his/her conception. And if the child is to be told, clearly there must be an assumption that the matter cannot be kept secret from other relatives and friends. In the light of this official advice, it might therefore be thought that couples more recently undertaking DI would be more likely to share information with significant others. This does not appear to be the case. Monach (1993), in his more recent study among DI couples, found that all couples had decided that as few people as possible should know about their recourse to DI treatment, and that the child would probably not be told. Monach records that the consultant responsible for these couples 'argued for encouraging openness about DI, particularly with the child. There was no evidence that the couples heard or heeded this view' (1993: 93). All available evidence points to the impression that the majority of couples have a strong inclination not to divulge their use of donor sperm.

Reasons for withholding information about DI

In discussions with family members one of the commonest reasons given for secrecy about the presence of a DI child in the family was merely a denial that there was any reason to tell. One man said: 'I keep on coming back to the fact that because it's successful I can't see any reason at all that anybody else needs to know.' This belief that there was no reason to tell was closely linked to the desire of the parents to present themselves as a 'normal' family, no different from any other. As one mother put it, 'We just want to carry on as though nothing has happened'. Secrecy allows a couple to deny DI. However, as Edwards points out 'Difference may be denied, but of course it is in denial that differentiation lies' (1993: 53).

This desire to appear as a 'normal' family points to the main reason why most couples think it best to keep DI secret; the fear of stigmatisation. One man said: 'I would find it very difficult to tell people, because it isn't so much the way I feel, I think it's the way other people would react. You can't rely on other people to be as thoughtful and understanding about problems as – well – as I am about my own problems.'

If their recourse to DI were known, many couples fear that their standing as a family would be diminished and that all members of the family would, in some way, be discredited. Stigma is seen not just to attach to the 'unnaturalness' of the DI procedure itself, but more importantly to the underlying condition of male infertility. Although infertility in general may be seen as stigmatising, it is apparent that male infertility is perceived to carry a greater stigma than infertility experienced by a woman. This differential stigma appears to be related to sex-role stereotypes. The male stereotype of 'head of the family' emerges in instrumental forms of behaviour and a man's infertility conflicts with this instrumental role. His inability to make his partner pregnant is incompatible with his socialised concept of appropriate masculine behaviour. He feels impotent in a social context even if he is not physically sexually impotent, and so concepts of infertility, impotency, lack of virility, and lack of masculinity become confused. Achilles (1993) argues that the practice of secrecy in DI is due, at least in part, to our inability to distinguish between the social meanings attached to reproduction and to sexuality, particularly in relation to male sexuality, male reproduction, and male infertility.

The other main reason underlying couples' preference for secrecy is that they are aware that DI holds important implications for family relationships. Their own parents would expect that any grandchildren would result from within the union between their respective son and daughter. Couples were aware that DI would create a situation of imbalance, with consanguineal or 'blood' relationships being present on the maternal side of the family which would be absent on the paternal side. However the major fear about relationships was that if the child became aware of his/her donor conception, the child's relationship with the parents, particularly the father, would be damaged. One father said quietly: 'I'd be afraid perhaps he might turn against me – I'd be afraid of that.'

The danger of accidental disclosure

Several decades ago, when the incidence and availability of DI was restricted, it may perhaps have been possible to keep the fact of DI secret from the children of the family. That possibility is now much less likely given the publicity which is afforded to the new reproductive technologies.

Adoption research has shown that accidental disclosure about a child's origins is much more likely to be damaging to family relationships than purposeful and planned disclosure. It would therefore appear to be in the best interests of the parents as well as the children conceived by DI that they should purposefully be made aware of their different origins before they learn of this in an accidental fashion.

During the second round of interviews with parents of young children conceived by DI, it was the parents' belief that none of their children had found out accidentally about their donor conception. The couples tended to be sanguine about the possibility of their children finding out from people who know, even when several friends and relatives had been told. Comments to the children such as, 'You've always been expensive, even before you were born', were seen as quite innocent. Several of the children knew their parents had had to seek medical help in order to conceive: 'She knows she's special – 'we had to wait three years for you' – but she doesn't know how, or anything.' One couple said that if comments about likeness were made 'We have a little private smile'. It is very likely that children are more aware that something lies behind such apparently hidden messages than parents suppose; as one mother said, 'children are very astute – they can hear things round corners'.

Despite the couples' belief that only specific known people are aware of their children's donor origins, it is of course impossible to say how many people actually know. Secrets are for telling and there is for most people an almost irresistible temptation to share a secret with at least one other confidant. The network of people who have been told at some time is likely to be much wider than parents think. Other children in the family, perhaps cousins, might well overhear conversations and then discuss what they have heard with the children concerned. Likewise there is no certainty about the parents' belief that the children do not know about, or suspect, their donor conception; they would be unlikely to confront their parents with such knowledge even if they did. Adoption research has shown that children who find out accidentally about their adopted status are often unable to discuss with their parents what they have learned. It would seem that the children are aware that acknowledging such information has the power to damage relationships and the cohesion of the family group. If the trauma of accidental disclosure is to be avoided there would appear to be strong pragmatic reasons in favour of making the child aware in a purposeful and planned way.

Support for information sharing among family members

There is little doubt that couples commencing DI are presented with confusing messages about the wisdom of sharing or withholding information.

Blyth asserts that 'recipients [of DI] have become pawns in the face of conflicting attitudes and advice concerning secrecy and openness. Broadly
speaking clinical practitioners tend to advocate secrecy (and occasionally
outright deception) whilst social workers and social scientists tend to advocate openness' (1991: 53). Although the official recommendations published by the RCOG (1992a and b) now encourage parents to consider
telling the child, it is clear that many practitioners are sceptical of the
wisdom of this advice and remain to be convinced that their traditional
commitment to secrecy is not more sensible. Here we see, in stark form,
differences in the perception of individuals and their needs. In providing DI
there is, on one hand, the 'medical treatment' approach which concentrates
on the 'treatment' of an individual and, on the other hand, there is the perception of the individual DI recipient and the resulting child in terms of a
set of family relationships. What makes this situation more complex from
the medical treatment perspective is that the fit mother is being treated in
order to create a family which, by definition, is primarily concerned with
relationships. It seems that the state of confusion is not confined to those
seeking DI 'treatment'.

One positive development in recent years has been the establishment of
self-help support groups for families where the parents wish to be more
open with their children. It would be dishonest, however, to suggest that
merely telling the child of his/her origins will solve all problems. Indeed, the
coming to terms with an absent biological link will have to be faced and
new problems might even be introduced. When DI is approached openly
and honestly, it is evident that any child so created will be in a position of
some disadvantage as he/she will know almost nothing of his/her genetic
father.

It remains anomalous that the identity of one of the prime actors in this
social creation of a family, the semen provider, is not to be known. Donor
anonymity is a legal requirement in the United Kingdom and disclosure of
a donor's identity could result in prosecution. Those providing the DI
service support the anonymous status of semen providers for pragmatic
reasons; they fear that their supply of donors would be much reduced if
anonymity were not ensured. Legislators support anonymity for a different
reason; they appear to see the anonymity of semen providers as a mechanism to protect the recipient family from intrusion by a third party
(Haimes 1990). Blyth (1991) points out that encouragement to openness in
a climate of service provision which requires donor anonymity appears to
be an example of double messages being given to vulnerable people.
Certainly many couples assert that if they cannot tell the child everything
then it is preferable to tell them nothing. The code of practice of the
Human Fertilisation and Embryology Authority makes provision for brief

non-identifying biographical details about the semen provider to be made available to recipient couples. However, this is not mandatory and there appears to be some confusion among clinicians about the purpose of this provision. It is not clear how great a priority is given to providing such information to couples, how much is passed on to the child, and how much understanding there is of the primary purpose of this information being for the child to know more of his/her background. Adoption research has shown that children benefit from knowing something about the story of their biological parents.

The research interviews confirmed that among couples who did not wish their children to know about their donor conception, donor anonymity was seen as a means of protecting the integrity of their family life in general and their role as parents in particular. Anonymity ensured there was no man in the background who might possess expectations about access to 'his' child. However, among parents who had told their children about their donor conception there was a firm but opposing belief that their children should be able to have access to information about the donor, even amounting to his identity. They believed that when their children were older they might quite reasonably wish to know about the donor and they should not be denied this information. Present legislation ensures that records are not destroyed; a central register of donors must be maintained. However, the Registrar is forbidden to divulge the identity of any donor, though he may give certain limited information (after counselling) to any 'child' conceived by DI who requests it on reaching the age of eighteen years.

Conclusion

Since human life began, human beings have developed arrangements and rules which regulate their relationships with each other. These relationships are often complex and appear impossible to disentangle into identifiable conceptual components that can be communicated easily to others for the purposes of meaningful discussion. What we do know about these relationships is that they possess a mixture of objective and identifiable characteristics which are intrinsically linked to other less identifiable characteristics of a vague, subjective kind based on the feelings, assumptions and intuition exhibited by the individual members of these groups. Among the most significant of these groupings there is one in which members appear to have particularly intimate and familiar relationships with each other. This familiarity is described also by objective characteristics relating to the definition of who reproduces by or with whom and by the subjective interpretations of these activities. Members of this 'familiar' group place a high value on the rights, duties and expectations of its members in relation to behaviour associated with reproduction and the care of new members of the family. Clearly the control of reproduction and the distribution of responsibilities relating to the care of family members has deep significance not only for the individual group members but also for the family group as a whole and, in turn, for the family's interaction with other family groups. This significance is demonstrated by the concern of others when these relationships go awry in some way as much as by manifest success in their functioning. Indeed, the complex make-up of these relationships has led to the situation whereby it is only when a dysfunction of some sort is apparent that the values of the underlying relationships can be glimpsed.

So it is with the situation where the biological and social dimensions of individual reproduction can be separated. It was not until the beginning of the twentieth century that reports were published describing for the first time the ability of human beings to reproduce in the absence of an act of sexual intercourse. This first description of DI drew attention to the creation of family relationships by males who were not able themselves to 'father' a child. The study of the meaning of family life among potential parents seeking DI to resolve their childlessness, and eventually among children created in this way, introduces an opportunity for examining the most enduring, yet mystifying, set of relationships in human experience.

NOTE

The authors wish to acknowledge funding received from the Economic and Social Research Council for the research project on which this chapter is based.

REFERENCES

Achilles, R. (1993) 'Protection from what? The secret life of donor insemination'. *Politics & the Life Sciences* 12(2): 171–2.

Blyth, E. (1991) *Infertility and assisted reproduction: practice issues for counsellors.* British Association of Social Workers, pp. 52–62.

Davis, K. (1984) 'The study of marriage and the family as a scientific discipline'. Paper presented to the American Sociological Association.

Eck-Menning, B. E. (1977) *Infertility: a guide for the childless couple.* Eaglewood Cliffs, NJ: Prentice Hall.

Edwards, J. (1993) 'Explicit connections: ethnographic enquiry in north-west England'. In: J. Edwards *et al.*, eds., *Technologies of Procreation: kinship in the age of assisted conception.* Manchester: Manchester University Press, pp. 42–66.

Haimes, E. (1990) 'Family Connections: the management of biological origins in the new reproductive technologies'. PhD thesis, University of Newcastle upon Tyne.

(1993) 'Secrecy and openness in donor insemination: a sociological comment on Daniels & Taylor'. *Politics & the Life Sciences* 12(2): 178–9.

52   Robert and Elizabeth Snowden

Hill, J. L. (1991) 'What does it mean to be a "parent"? The claims of biology as the basis for parental rights'. *New York University Law Review* 66: 353–420.

Holmes, H. B. (1993) 'Openness, fatherhood, and responsibility: a feminist analysis'. *Politics & the Life Sciences* 12(2): 180–2.

Human Fertilisation and Embryology Act 1990. United Kingdom Government.

Kubler-Ross, E. (1969) *On death and dying*. New York: Macmillan.

Lauritzen, P. (1993) *Pursuing parenthood: ethical issues in assisted reproduction*. Bloomington: Indiana University Press.

Lindahl, M. and Back, K. (1987) 'Lineage identity and generational continuity: family history and family reunions'. *Comparative Gerontology* B1: 30–4.

McNeil, M. (1990) 'Reproductive technologies: a new terrain for the sociology of technology'. In M. McNeil *et al.*, eds., *The new reproductive technologies*. Basingstoke: Macmillan.

McWhinnie, A. M. (1993) 'Doubts and realities in DI family relationships'. *Politics & the Life Sciences* 12(2): 189–91.

Mays, A. (1994) 'Personal view on donor insemination'. *Issue* Winter, p. 7.

Monach, J. H. (1993) *Childless: no choice. The experience of involuntary childlessness*. London: Routledge.

O'Brien, M. (1981) *The politics of reproduction*. New York: Routledge & Kegan Paul.

Radcliffe-Brown, A. and Forde, D., eds. (1950). *African systems of kinship and marriage*. Oxford: Oxford University Press.

RCOG Fertility Committee (1992) *Infertility: guidelines for practice*. London: RCOG.

RCOG (1992) *Donor insemination: patient information booklet*. London: RCOG.

Snowden, R. and Snowden, E. (1991) End of Award Report to ESRC Ref. R000 23 1651.

(1993) *The gift of a child: revised edition*, Exeter: University of Exeter Press.

(1994) 'A research programme in the UK to assess the social and psychological implications of the use of donor insemination to alleviate childlessness'. In L. J. Severy, ed., *Advances in population*. London: Jessica Kingsley, vol. 2, pp. 89–118.

Snowden, R., Mitchell, G. D. and Snowden, E. M. (1983) *Artificial reproduction: a social investigation*. London: Allen & Unwin.

Triseliotis, J. (1993) 'Donor insemination and the child'. *Politics and the Life Sciences*, 12(2): 195–7.

Warnock, M. (1984) *Report of the Committee of Inquiry into Human Fertilisation & Embryology*, London: HMSO.

4 The making of 'the DI child': changing representations of people conceived through donor insemination

Erica Haimes

Introduction

The purpose of donor insemination is starkly simple: to create a child. However, since surprisingly little is known about the babies conceived in this way, it is not possible to present a view of DI from the child's perspective, since we do not really know what that is. What we do know comes mostly from what the other parties involved in DI (e.g. the clinicians, the recipients, the policymakers, the social analysts) consider to be the child's needs and interests.

In this chapter I shall examine how others have represented the 'DI child', in both senses of 'representation': how others have claimed to speak on behalf of the 'child' and how, in making such claims, they have also presented a certain image of DI offspring and have shaped how they might be perceived. The 'DI child' is as much, if not more, a product of these social processes as s/he is of the physiological. I shall use extensive quotations from various sources as a way of displaying the data from which my interpretations have been drawn, to show how such representations have varied over time.

Elsewhere I have written about the practical, clinical and policy issues around the 'DI child' (e.g. Haimes 1990, 1992, 1993) but here I want to provide an analysis at another level, that focuses not so much on the issues themselves but on what those issues reveal about the way in which the person conceived by DI is seen by others. By taking such a step back we can see that the issues that are usually presented on the DI child do not simply mirror the world of DI but in fact contribute to the process whereby that world is actively constructed and packaged by those participating in it. Thus, I am less concerned to try to establish what does or ought to happen to or for DI adults, as I am to review the claims that others make about what does or ought to happen, in order to see what the claims themselves reveal about the way in which the DI person is seen.

In the final section of the chapter I shall address a third level of representation: that of self-representation, by reviewing the little that is known about

53

how people conceived by DI see themselves. This provides the bare beginnings of what might be labelled 'the DI adults' perspective' (though there is no reason to suppose that one single voice will emerge) as well as the opportunity to draw comparisons between the three types of representations.

The DI child: name and number?

Before going further, two other points need to be considered. First, what to call people conceived through DI? So far, I have deliberately used a range of labels: 'child', 'children', 'babies', 'people conceived through DI'. Others have used phrases such as 'a donated child' (Barton *et al.* 1945), 'the AID child' (Brandon 1979) and, more provocatively, 'custom-made child' (Holmes *et al.* 1981) and 'turkey-baster babies' (Stephenson and Wagner 1991).[1] More recently, the terms 'offspring' and 'donor offspring' have been used.

This proliferation of labels goes to the heart of the issue of representation. For example, the labelling of such people as 'babies' can suggest that they are to be seen as merely the end-product of DI, whereas labelling them 'children', 'offspring', 'adults', 'people' can suggest that they have lives and biographies with the potential to extend beyond their origins in DI.

I shall tend to use the label 'people conceived by DI'.[2] Though clumsy, this has two advantages: first, it situates this group in relation to the practice of DI rather than to any other party (recipients, donors etc); second, it follows the trend of favouring phrases such as 'People with AIDS' and 'people with disabilities',[3] which are more open-ended and which place the person first before qualifying him/her as a particular type of person.[4] Of course, the choice of one label over others does not resolve the debate: it simply establishes another claim.

A second aspect to consider is the number of people conceived by DI. This would be a standard scene-setting step to make but discussions about numbers are similar to discussions about labels: more revealing of the assumptions underpinning DI than of the 'facts'. Nobody knows how many people have been conceived through DI. Indeed, even those of us writing or reading this book are unlikely to know if we are to be counted amongst their number.[5]

We are beginning to get more accurate assessments as recently established record-keeping documents the number of times DI is used, the number of users and the expected success rate. Achilles (1992) reviews the somewhat fragmentary data: one survey suggested there were 30,000 births in the United States from DI in 1986–87 and that the total population conceived by DI in the United States is more than 1,000,000; France reports approximately 1,700 DI births per annum, with a total population of

16,000; Australia reports a DI birth rate of approximately 2,000 per annum; Switzerland and the Netherlands report more than 1,000 per annum; Sweden more than 300 per annum; Japan has an estimated DI population of 10,000. Achilles suggests these figures are underestimates, so clearly the number of people actually born from DI is not insignificant.

Does this uncertainty matter? What more would we learn about the experience of being conceived by DI if we had this knowledge? The usual reasons for trying to count the numbers affected by any issue are: to see how widespread the experience is (does it affect a minority or a majority of people?); to see if there are any patterns amongst those affected (e.g. of age, ethnicity, class) and to start to judge how important the issue might be from a socio-political or policy-making point of view. This then contributes to the cultural characterisations of the people involved.

In the case of people conceived by DI it may be that the lack of knowledge of numbers contributes to their cultural characterisation.[6] For example, they may be viewed as 'different' simply because it is assumed that they are few in number. Alternatively, since we know so little about the prevalence of the practice and since we cannot tell by looking, any one of us might have been conceived by DI. Both characterisations (as 'other' or as 'any one of us') derive their cultural significance from the awareness that in most Euro-American societies, it is not a trivial point to be conceived using the gametes of someone other than the adults raising you as your parents. Thus we want to know which of us has the likelihood of being a member of that category. Therefore, it does 'matter' how many people have been conceived by DI, but it 'only' matters because this interest rests upon a more pervasive, culturally significant interest in social and biological relationships (see chapter 8 by Edwards in this collection).

It would be possible to spend the whole chapter on just these two points. They are indicative of a more general difficulty that will be apparent as we go through the chapter: how and where to locate those who have been conceived by DI within the social relationships around DI?

A brief history of 'the DI child'

We can begin to study the changing representations of the person conceived by DI by returning to the 'first story of DI', describing an insemination that had occurred in 1884 (see chapter 6 by Novaes). The story describes events as turning full circle when the author, twenty-five years later in 1909 'shook the hand' of the young man who had been conceived (Achilles 1992: 15–16). It is assumed that he, like his mother, remained ignorant of the process of conception. Quite what he made of the stranger's (presumably fulsome) handshake is unknown.

That account set a trend for the part that people conceived by DI played in early medical accounts of DI: as a successful outcome of a slightly risky (morally, physiologically, legally) procedure and ultimately therefore as an end which justified the means. Barton *et al.* (1945) provide one of the earliest examples of this: the person conceived is seen predominantly through the eyes and needs of the parents.

One has to bear in mind that the legal father may hope for a donated child with whose personality he might be in accord, and it must further be remembered that difficulties in the father-son relationship might be accentuated by the circumstances of A.I.D. Obviously, even the most careful choice of the donor for each case could not guarantee the desired characteristics, but it would increase the chances of matching parent and child. (1945: 41)

In this article, the few direct implications for 'the child' that are mentioned are seen to arise from the procedures of DI itself, but there is no mention, for example, of how the 'child' will make sense of the circumstances of his/her conception.

This style of treating the person conceived through DI as an end product was not common to all accounts of DI however. In the United Kingdom Barton's article prompted a response from the archbishop of Canterbury who commissioned a report on DI. Here the image of the DI 'child' was significantly different to that presented in Barton's article. The commission worried about the effect on the 'child' of knowing the method of conception: 'With the AID child there are, in this respect, manifest difficulties. The necessary explanations might inflict severe psychological injury and increase insecurity' (1948: 26–7). Not the least of these was the stigma of illegitimacy. On the other hand the commission questioned the attitude of doctors and parents who thought that, since family life appeared settled and 'the episode of insemination soon becomes unimportant', the 'child' would 'not need to be told of his origins' (1948: 27). In trying to substantiate such claims, the commission soon discovered that, 'the element of secrecy involved prohibits observation on scientific lines and the publication of findings' (1948: 29).

This secrecy, plus the associated problems of adultery and illegitimacy (Haimes 1990), led the legal experts to recommend the criminalisation of DI. The commission concluded that DI 'defrauds the child begotten and deceives both his putative kinsmen and society at large . . . For the child there must always be the risk of disclosure, deliberate or unintended, of the circumstances of his conception' (1948: 58). For the commission therefore DI was a damaging way to be conceived, but secrecy only compounded the difficulties and was itself the strongest indicator of the undesirability of the practice.

The commission displayed extensive concern for the 'child's' position, but this was less central to two other reports that figure prominently in the UK history of DI. The Feversham Committee (1958–1960) was asked to consider whether the interests of individuals and society warranted any changes in the law on artificial insemination (Haimes 1990). They considered that to be conceived in this way could only be a 'handicap'. This view was compounded by uncertainties about what was inherited from 'an unknown third person' and the likelihood of damaged family relationships through the suppression of the truth about the 'child's' conception. Under a section entitled 'The Effect on the Child of Hearing of his Origin', the committee suggested difficulties would arise from the 'child' learning of his/her conception by accident: (a) that his/her 'parents' had deceived him/her; (b) that s/he was illegitimate and (c) that s/he was conceived 'through a test-tube, a method of conception which is at the present time repugnant to a considerable section of the community' (1960: 45). On the other hand, they did not feel that the child should be told how s/he was conceived:

we are not convinced that this course would as a rule be in the child's best interests. The effect on the child might be, broadly speaking, the same as if he were to hear of the matter by accident, except that he would know that his 'parents' had not intended that he should be permanently deceived. No doubt if the relationship between him, his mother and her husband were a happy one and the explanation of his origin was managed with tact and understanding, the emotional impact of the news would be considerably lessened. But, whatever the circumstances of their revelation, the facts could scarcely be other than disturbing. (1960: 46)

They recommended 'that in the interests of the child alone . . . the practice should be discouraged' (1960: 46) and they hoped that this recommendation alone would be enough to ensure the disappearance of DI.

The Peel Report (1973) was produced by a panel established in 1971 by the British Medical Association in response to an increasing number of enquiries for information about DI. In contrast to the earlier reports this report said very little about how information relating to the 'child's' origins should be handled. The panel favoured follow-up studies of DI families, despite being urged to reject these, because they wanted to know about the impact of DI on families and about the long-term genetic effects on the 'children'. There was no mention of whether they felt the 'child' should be told of his/her conception, nor even of the general secrecy surrounding DI.

This brief history (1945–1973), although taken from just one country, gives a reasonable idea of the range of different ways in which the person conceived by DI could be perceived. The Archbishop's Commission, the Feversham Committee and Barton all felt that it would be damaging for a 'child' to be identified as having been conceived by DI. However, whilst the clinicians expressed the view, explicitly in Barton and implicitly in the Peel Report, that this could be resolved by keeping the 'child's' origins secret, the Archbishop's Commission and the Feversham Committee felt that such secrecy was itself harmful, to families and to society, and was further reason for abandoning the practice of DI altogether.

It is possible to see from this material two strands in the history of DI and the representation of the 'child'; strands which are likely to have been apparent in other countries too. In the two key medical reports (Barton and Peel) the person conceived was seen as a successful outcome of an increasingly successful medical procedure, whereas in the other two reports the 'child' was seen (albeit still as a child) in a broader context, in terms of his/her future relationships with the nurturing parents and in terms of his/her image in the wider society.

This broader perspective gradually became characterised in the United Kingdom, the United States, Australia and elsewhere in terms of a concern with 'roots' and with 'origins'. If the 'child' understood these aspects about him/herself, it was reasoned, s/he would be able to deal with other aspects of having been conceived through DI (especially as concerns about the stigma of illegitimacy, in particular, were beginning to fade). In the late 1970s-early 1980s the focus on 'roots' as a way of representing the needs of the 'DI child' was consolidated. In 1980, George Annas, an American Professor of Law and Medicine, wrote:

Because of the current secrecy surrounding the practice of artificial insemination by donor, there are an estimated 250,000 children conceived by AID (at the rate of 6,000–10,000 annually in the United States) who will never be able to find their biological roots. There are almost no data available on these children, their psychological development, or their family life. The entire procedure has been shrouded in secrecy . . . most of the informal 'policies' concerning AID as it is currently practised in the United States have come about because of an exaggeration of potential legal pitfalls and a failure to pay sufficient attention to the best interests of the AID child. (1980: 331)

The above quotation neatly encapsulates the features of the 'roots' perspective: people conceived by DI were characterised as children; ideas about origins and roots were tied to those of biology (and, later, genetics); lack of information about origins was tied to the secrecy of DI practice; the lack of knowledge about the children conceived was seen as a failing, and, finally, the interests of other parties were seen as leading to a neglect of the 'child's' interests.[7] Cushan (1984) shows that very similar arguments were being made in Australia.

In the same article Annas tied the concern to protect and promote the 'child's' interests in DI to similar developments in adoption, and to the stimulus provided by the novel 'Roots'. It is worth noting that these observations were made by someone who could be considered an outsider to DI practice, with no interests to protect. The growing commentary on DI by others not directly involved as doctors, recipients and donors was a feature of the 1980s that had a major impact on the way in which the 'DI child' was perceived.

Adoption researchers argued that adoption and DI experienced the same problems around secrecy, but could also benefit, therefore, from the same solutions of openness (Holland 1971; Brandon and Warner 1977; McWhinnie 1982). A growing awareness that adoptees reaching adulthood were increasingly expressing unhappiness with past secrecy had led to changes in practice:

On the basis of this adoption experience we recommend that serious account should be taken of the possibility that AID adults will have a similar desire for true knowledge of their origins and will wish to be reared by parents who do not deceive them on this score. (British Agencies for Adoption and Fostering Medical Group 1984: 11)

Openness in DI, they argued, involves telling the 'child' about the donation and providing positive details about the donor, but donor anonymity could be retained if that were needed to reassure donors and to keep them donating.

Another particularly influential body of work in the early 1980s that increased awareness of the 'DI child' in the United Kingdom, was produced by Snowden and colleagues (1981; 1983; see also chapter 3 in this collection). It was clear to them that, whatever was claimed to the contrary, the 'child's' interests were regarded as far less important than the social father's interests in keeping his infertility secret.

It is this deception connected with paternity which is the source of all secrecy surrounding the practice of AID. It could be said that keeping the child in ignorance of its genetic origin, ensuring the donor remains anonymous, undertaking the AID process in a clandestine atmosphere and even keeping the fact of AID from friends, neighbours and relatives stem from this fundamental issue of paternity. (1981: 94)

The importance of this body of work emerging in the 1970s-80s is not that it provided unproblematic solutions,[8] but rather that it was part of a wider period of transition for DI whereby the practice itself came more fully on to the public agenda (as much as anything because IVF and other forms of assisted conception had grabbed the public's and politicians' attention too) and other professionals, besides doctors, became involved in the field. This particular group of professionals, with experience in adoption and child care more generally, ensured that discussions around DI opened up to include and take account of the 'child'. Studies such as those from adoption then became part of the process of the social construction of the 'DI child'. They lent specialist professional authority to the concerns expressed earlier by the Archbishop's Commission and the Feversham Committee, by drawing upon theories of psychological need and development, informed variously by Freud, Piaget, Erikson, as well as by Sants' notion of 'genealogical bewilderment' (Humphrey and Humphrey 1986). The image that emerged from these influences was of a child at risk from impaired mental health unless steps were taken to ensure that s/he experienced as near normal psychological development as possible: a notion which itself was tied to ideas of the 'normal' development of 'identity'. This notion of identity was seen as rooted in ideas about the necessary knowledge of biological and genetic origins.

These studies also extended and clarified (though did not resolve) the debate over whether to tell the 'child' how s/he was conceived. By the late 1970s-early 1980s, three views were apparent on what the 'DI child' needed to know about his/her conception: first, the dominant view, propounded particularly by clinicians, was that s/he should be told absolutely nothing about the means of conception, let alone about the donor; a second view emerging from some adoption professionals was to tell the 'child' about the means of conception but nothing about the donor; a third view, from other adoption writers, was to be completely open to the 'child' about the means of conception and about the identity of the donor.

In the early 1980s this debate extended beyond the professional sphere into the policymaking forum, as a number of different countries attempted to review systematically the full range of developments in assisted conception. DI was included in most of these reviews and the question of how to manage the information about the 'child's' origins was a common theme, albeit one that was resolved in a variety of ways. In Australia, the Waller Report (1982–1984) said a less secretive approach would be better for the 'child', both in terms of emotional development and for ensuring better record-keeping, to allow medical information to be passed between the donors, parents and children and to allow for follow-up studies of the children. In Sweden, efforts were made to consider DI from the 'child's' perspective. It was argued that the 'child' had a right to know his/her origins, so legislation was passed in 1985 allowing that child, when adolescent or older, access to identifying information about the donor. The Swedish policy committee argued that

The basic consideration underlying the Committee's recommendations on artificial inseminations is the best interests of the child. If AID is considered from the viewpoint of the prospective child, there are weighty reasons in favour of a decision – despite the risk that in an initial stage the activity would decrease in hospitals – to demand that only such sperm donors are used who do not oppose that their identity may subsequently be disclosed to the child. (1983: 42/15)

In Germany the Benda Report (1985) recommended that the 'child' at age sixteen should have access to identifying information about the donor. In the United Kingdom the Warnock Committee argued that the more encompassing secrecy surrounding DI should be discouraged for the sake of the family and for the sake of the 'child'. They recommended that the importance to the 'child' of possessing genetic knowledge should be under-lined by providing him/her with 'basic information about the donor's ethnic origin and genetic health' at the age of eighteen (1984: 25). The donor would remain anonymous although 'We recognise that one consequence of this provision would be that AID children, even if informed about the cir-cumstances of their conception would never be entitled to know the iden-tity of their genetic fathers' (1984: 25).

By the mid-1980s, therefore, in those countries where DI was scrutinised (Walters 1987) the person conceived was a central part of how DI was debated, at both a professional and a political level. The issue of the 'child's' origins was seen as something that had to be dealt with and the focus became 'what to tell the child?'. The different responses to this question were each presented and defended in terms of the 'child's' best interests, defined by invoking vignettes in which the child would suffer as a conse-quence of the mishandling of the information concerning his/her origins. For example, 'it's better not to tell the child anything because of the stigma of illegitimacy' or 'it's better to tell the child because of the problems arising from family secrets' or 'it's better to tell the child everything about the donation and the donor because everyone has the need to know their genetic origins'. It was not possible to arbitrate between these different positions since they each invoked the same underlying claim. As we shall see, this claim gained further prominence as the child's welfare became a central part of the debates around assisted conception in the 1990s.

The 'DI child' in the 1990s

In the 1990s the debate over 'what to tell the child' continues, but it has been joined by three other issues that also focus on the 'child': the risks of inher-iting a genetic disease through a DI conception; the growing call for follow-up studies of children conceived by DI, and, how best to protect the welfare of the child.

As a brief update on the origins issue, Austria has followed the Swedish model by legislating for access to identifying information about the donor by the 'child' (Morgan and Bernatt 1992). Australia allows for access to identifying information about the donor if he gives his agreement in writing at the time of the request. In the United Kingdom and in Canada the 'child' can gain access to non-identifying information at the age of eighteen. In

New Zealand there have been various moves towards identifying donors to the recipients (Adair 1994) and 'children', through the notion of 'good professional practice', rather than through formal legislation (Daniels 1995). In Belgium, Spain and France, donor anonymity is still the norm.

The risks to the 'child' of inheriting genetically transmitted diseases from the donor has emerged as an important issue in the 1990s. Since the elimination of all risks is unlikely given current knowledge, the question becomes 'what is the acceptable risk?' (Novaes 1994: 98) and consequently how are the interests of the person conceived represented?

As an example, the 1990 American Fertility Society guidelines state that the purpose of screening donors is to protect recipient women from sexually transmitted diseases and to protect the resultant children from genetically transmitted diseases. The guidelines suggest a 'minimal genetic screen' for a number of conditions, from: 'nontrivial malformations' (e.g. spina bifida), which have up to a 5 per cent chance of occurring in the child of an affected man; 'non trivial mendelian disorders' (e.g. haemophilia) which have a 50 per cent chance of appearing in the man's child, and familial diseases with a genetic component (e.g. diabetes) which 'represent an appreciable risk for the child, which would range from 50 per cent to 15 per cent' (1990: 8S).

Comments by the Chairman of the AFS suggest the balance of concern lies with the recipient woman.

Because HIV is a potentially fatal illness and hepatitis and other STDs are severely debilitating it is essential to protect the recipient against these infections. According to a report from the Office of Technology Assessment some 30,000 infants are conceived in the United States each year by women inseminated with donor sperm. The protection of these women and their offspring must be the prime concern of all professionals providing AID service. (1990: 400)

The British Andrology Society fully endorsed the AFS guidelines, but in a way that shifted, on paper at least, the balance of concern to the people conceived by DI: 'The aims of these guidelines are limited specifically to the protection of the offspring of donor insemination treatment from heritable genetic disorders and the offspring and recipient women from infection' (1993: 1521).

The point here is not to claim that these two reports represent significant differences in practice or attitudes between the two societies, nor the two countries, but to show how the person conceived by DI can be represented in two very different ways, even when the detailed substantive content and context is almost exactly the same. This brief snapshot shows once again the dilemma that clinicians have in formulating their view of the 'DI child'. Clearly the woman is at risk every time she receives semen whilst a 'child' is only at risk if s/he is actually conceived. On the other hand, clinicians have to take precautions to protect the 'child' in every individual treatment, in case it results in a conception. Thus, whilst the woman is unambiguously present, the person conceived is both there and not there; with a potential presence in the future but requiring attention as if present now.

It could be argued that the person conceived tends to be seen in this ambivalent way because there have been very few studies of them, despite the duration of established DI practice. Hence there is little sense of them as fully-formed, adult human beings. This, it will be remembered, was one of the complaints made by Annas in 1980. Studies by Iizuka (1968) in Japan, Langer (1969) in Israel and Leeton and Blackwell (1982) reported on the physical and psychological developments of children conceived by DI, but these were each very small, narrow, isolated studies, which together convey only a very fragmented sense of the children's experiences (Haimes 1990). It is not really surprising that so few follow-up studies have been conducted, since most doctors would have been contradicting their own advice and practice if they had attempted to persuade 'successful' couples to allow their DI children to be subjects in such a study.

However, the development of other techniques of assisted conception, most notably IVF, has led to interest in the psychological and physical development of all the children conceived, initially because of uncertainty about the long-term effects of manipulating gametes and intervening with the process of fertilisation. This, alongside the already documented gradual relaxation of views around the secrecy of DI, has made a systematic follow-up of DI children (if not yet adults) at least comtemplatable. Golombok *et al.* (1995) report one of the first attempts. This UK study investigated both the quality of the parenting and the childrens' 'psychiatric state' in families created through DI and IVF: these were then compared with families with a 'naturally' conceived child and with adoptive families. Forty-five DI children, four to eight years old, were included in the study. None had been told about their method of conception. The evidence showed that 'for children aged 4–8 years at least, keeping the method of conception secret from the child does not appear to have a negative impact on family relationships' (1995: 297). The researchers acknowledged: 'It is yet to be seen how many parents will decide to tell the children as they grow up, and whether difficulties will arise as issues of identity become more salient at adolescence' (1995: 297). This study reflects issues that have arisen hitherto but also represents a significant development from that past. The links lie in the way that the children are presented: as vehicles for the measurement of normal and abnormal development (physical, psychological, familial) rather than as active, sense-making social actors in their own right. Also the focus on the child obscures the fact that there are numerous fully-adult DI people who could provide a much broader perspective: if only they and the researchers knew who they were.

On the other hand, this study is a further indication of the changes in the way that DI is perceived: it is now possible for the concerns that led to the study to be sufficiently acknowledged, for a large-scale research project to be conducted, with an expectation that the relevant parties (in particular, DI recipients) would participate. That the research could be contemplated and conducted is more significant, in terms of the cultural history of DI, than the actual findings.

Another strand of discussion has emerged in the 1990s: the concern with the 'welfare of the child'. This is important because it is part of the distinctive framework of contemporary views on assisted conception and because it can be used to counter the suggestion that concern with the genetic risks to the 'child' and with his/her psychological and physical development amounts to little more than a concern to prove that DI has a successful outcome. To test this out, however, we need to see what is meant by the phrase 'the welfare of the child', how it emerged and what it means in relation to DI.

The UK Human Fertilisation and Embryology Act, 1990 states that 'a woman shall not be provided with treatment services unless account has been taken of the welfare of any child who may be born as a result of the treatment (including the need of that child for a father) and of any child who may be affected by the birth' (HFE Act, 1990: S13, 5). This applies to DI, egg and embryo donation and to IVF. Lieberman *et al.* (1994), who conducted a survey amongst practitioners on the workings of the act, report that 'the ambiguities and practical difficulties relating to "the need to take into account the welfare of any child born or existing children . . ."' before providing licensed treatment gave cause for comment and concern' (1994: 1781).

Shenfield (1994a) suggests there are 'cultural differences . . . in the interpretation of the welfare or best interests of the child' (1994a: 1352), citing the contrast between 'the compulsory information of their genetic origin to children born of sperm donation in Sweden when reaching adulthood . . . and . . . the restrictive German law forbidding oocyte and embryo donation . . .' (1994a: 1352). In France, she says, '[the] welfare of the child is considered to be best served if he/she is born to a couple (which in French law means heterosexual couple) who also should be of reproductive age' (1994a: 1353). Thus these newer strands of concern for the child combine with, rather than replace, longer-established debates, on information about origins.

Englert (1994), writing from a fertility unit in Belgium, expresses concern that 'the welfare of the child' can be used either to oppose reproductive technologies generally or to oppose the use of DI by single women. Englert's clinic offers DI to both single women and homosexual couples. The grounds for being accepted for treatment are based

essentially on the existence of a solid relationship network surrounding the enquirers, on their perception of the very special nature of the project and their caution with regard to the potential difficulties facing the child. Their capacity to verbalize and to explain their plans for the child is also taken into account. (1994: 1970)

This constitutes for Englert sufficient consideration for the welfare of the child. Golombok and Tasker (1994) conclude from their review of the literature that 'existing research on lesbian and single-parent families does not indicate that these children would be at risk for psychological problems' (1994: 1975). Shenfield (1994), though, requires evidence to show that homosexual couples or single women can provide a family 'at least as good as the imperfect' heterosexual family, before being convinced that the welfare of 'the most vulnerable part in the reproductive equation, the potential child' is being suitably protected (1994b: 1977).

Clearly this discussion will continue. For our interests in this chapter the important point to note is that the 'welfare of the child' is a complex matter that goes beyond the question of what a person conceived by DI might need, to raising more general questions about the sorts of people suitable to receive DI, to yet wider questions about the social and political acceptability of different family forms. This reminds us that questions about people conceived by DI are not separable from wider issues. As Englert observes, 'the appeal to the notion of "the interests of the child" has to be handled with the greatest care. It has, throughout all debates in reproductive medicine, served many causes . . .' (1994: 1970).[9] The 'welfare of the child' is particularly vulnerable to being used as a banner under which to rally all sorts of causes because there has been very sparse information from people conceived by DI themselves. Had they had a voice it might have been possible at least to add their own views on what they would consider to be their best interests: not that they would necessarily constitute the only authoritative voice in this debate but they would at least be a voice that would require attention.

Representations of people conceived by DI: by themselves

The question to which we now turn is how the representations given by others compare with what DI people themselves consider to be their own image and interests. The voices heard here are unlikely to be representative of all DI people, given their small number. Indeed, it could be argued that they are highly atypical, if only because they know how they were conceived.[10] None the less, they provide a chance to see other images, and to hear other views: much can be learnt from these directly and from comparing them to the images and views expressed in this chapter hitherto.

Donors' Offspring was founded in 1982 in America by Candace Turner[11] who had been conceived by DI in 1948 and had tried to find out about the donor's medical and cultural history. Having had difficulty in doing this she launched a campaign for the right for all DI-conceived people to know about their origins and to prevent the abuse of DI practice. In a document entitled, 'The kind of parents all AID children would like to have' (nd), Turner argues that a DI child would want 'parents who plan to tell them the facts of their conception before they reach 12 years of age . . . We hope our parents will get detailed information either sealed or unsealed for us to read later of our medical, cultural and character backgrounds from the donor (nd: 2). She provides a model bedtime story, to assist parents in telling a four-year-old child of his/her conception and suggests developments in the story as the child gets older. Once the child is thirteen–sixteen years old, Turner suggests s/he should be given all known information, except the donor's name which should be made available either when s/he reaches eighteen or earlier if something happens to his/her parents. Pictures of the donor should be provided. She suggests that donors could be relatives of the husband and have a 'favourite uncle' role. The other possibility she suggests is for several of the husband's friends or relatives to donate, with only the doctor, and eventually the 'child', after the age of eighteen, knowing whose sperm was actually used.

Turner claims that when information has been given,

Grandparents and offspring and others took the news well, rarely referred to it again, yet seemed to be happy to be trusted with the information. Many offspring felt proud and closer to their parents. Some were relieved to know their Dad's diseases would not threaten their futures and cause subfertility . . . (1982: 4)

Since Turner's campaign others have called for similar rights. Achilles concludes that the experiences of five DI adults that she interviewed 'illustrate most clearly that secrecy is not only sometimes infeasible but definitely not beneficial' (1986: 115). However it should be noted that out of these five people one was Candy Turner, another was her brother, a third was Suzanne Rubin (see below); three wanted to find out more information, two did not.

Robert Snowden also spoke with a small number of people whose parents had told them of their DI conception.

It may be significant that the young people . . . had all been told in a purposeful and planned way. These young adults had accepted their AID status equably and none of them had found it a particularly traumatic experience. They had certainly been surprised when they were told, but some of that surprise was because their parents had kept the matter such a close secret for so many years. None of them regretted the fact they had been conceived by AID. They were enjoying life and happy to be alive and realised that they owed their existence to AID. They were also pleased to feel that their parents had wanted a child so badly, and that they were that child who had fulfilled their parents' wishes. (1990: 82)

They were not 'overly curious' about the donor, 'nor did they have a feeling of lack of identity themselves, or a sense of not being sure who they were' (1990: 82). Snowden concludes that fears expressed by DI recipients about openness were likely to be unfounded.

An article in the *New York Times Magazine* (Orenstein 1995) contrasted various cases, the first of which concerned Suzanne Ariel who, as Suzanne Rubin, had published an account of what it was like to discover she had been conceived through DI. Ariel referred to the 'dirty secret' of DI in her family, compounded by another secret, that she herself, aged fifteen, had surrendered a baby for adoption. It was her attempts to contact the adoptive family that led her father to tell her that she had been conceived through DI. Her reaction had been 'Goddammit, I knew it!' and she decided to try to track down the donor. After three years of searching she saw a picture of her parents' DI doctor and was forced to conclude that he had used his own semen: 'It was like looking at a picture of myself . . . The arrogance of that man! The deceit! My parents trusted him' (1995: 35). Another DI adult, Bill Cordray, had been told of his conception when he confessed to his mother that he suspected her of having had an affair and becoming pregnant with him: 'It was the only explanation I could come up with' for the distance between him and his father. He regrets the secrecy:

In a normal family, the dad may be distanced for other reasons . . . because of personality or whatever. But this threw an extra element in that was pathological. Knowing my Dad's capacity for love, I feel things would have been better if everything had been open. At least there would have been a better chance. (Orenstein 1995: 32)

Having experienced difficulty getting information about the donor he started to feel he had no right to it: until he heard a DI practitioner on the radio: 'This guy was talking about their marvellous policies on secrecy and how the donors will never meet the child . . . It made me angry . . . This guy's arrogance blew me away. Suddenly I thought, "What do you mean, I have no rights?"' (1995: 35). He also came to suspect that his parents' physician had been the donor, but then wondered if the physician had himself made use of the same donor as Bill's parents, having discovered a striking resemblance between himself and the physician's son. His younger brother had also been conceived by DI but their mother did not want him to be told: 'She thought Jeff was too young to know the truth – he was 28 – and I couldn't understand why she'd keep it a secret from him . . . Because it wasn't a shock to me to find out. The shock was that they'd waited so damn long . . . it was cruel. I had to tell him' (1995: 32). Bill's brother 'admits that he's never felt much interest in tracking down his own donor father . . . "I'm curious but not to the point of being obsessed with it"' (1995: 50).

Orenstein then draws a further contrast between Ariel and Cordray on the one hand and a group of three young brothers, who had all been conceived using semen from the same donor. Their parents had been treated at the Sperm Bank of California which has an identity-release programme, meaning that adults conceived by DI can, once they are eighteen, obtain the names, addresses, social security numbers, driving licence numbers and telephone numbers of the donors. The oldest boy in the family 'explains what he knows about the circumstances of his birth. "We're from a sperm bank", the ten-year-old says, matter-of-factly. Before turning back to the TV, he adds that he'd like to meet the man someday: "It would be cool"' (1995: 58). Orenstein describes this last family as 'the very model of the next-wave donor insemination family' (1995: 58), implying both approval of their attitude and also an inexorable progression towards greater openness.

To talk so confidently of a 'next wave' is perhaps overstating a claim for changes in practice that are by no means all moving in the same direction, as we have seen elsewhere in this chapter. Also it is quite evident that those conceived by DI express a range of views and experience a range of reactions, both between individuals and within the same person at different points in their lives. The person conceived by DI is not a single entity, speaking with one voice and expressing one set of needs. The claims made by other parties about, and on behalf of, the 'DI child', need to be judged in the light of this finding.

Conclusions

We can see from the material presented here that the person conceived plays a very important part in the DI story and that this part has been characterised in many different ways, in terms of their needs, their interests and who and what they are. There are two broad and recurrent tendencies in these characterisations. First, the tendency to see the person conceived not so much as an individual but as the end result of the DI procedure, towards which many actions are directed and efforts devoted. In this perspective the person conceived is seen as a measure of success for DI as a whole: DI works because it produces a baby. This is perhaps most obvious in the 'first story' of DI and in Barton's article from 1945, but it is just as much a part of later developments too.

A second[12] tendency is to see the person conceived as a child, which to some extent counters the view of the baby as the end result of DI. Mere reference to children and childhood indicates that there are all sorts of other events and relationships that follow on from the successful birth. For this child, the DI conception is considered significant in terms of his/her origins, but equally the child is viewed as having moved beyond that stage, and as developing in other ways.

These different representations have come to the fore at different points in the history of DI. Whilst it might be argued that it is preferable to see the person conceived as a child, rather than as a measure of success, and then (but even more so) as an adult, it is in fact not my intention to suggest that there has been a smooth progression from one, less enlightened to other, more enlightened, representations, nor even to suggest that there ought to be this 'progression'. Rather I hope to have shown how all these different representations emerge from different sources and overlap and mingle at different times. The significance of these representations is not that they show a particular development in how people conceived by DI are perceived, but that as representations, they tell us more about DI as a whole, since they reflect, and help to constitute, the wider network of social relationships that surround the practice of DI.

For example, the tendency to see the person conceived as a measure of the successful outcome of DI practice resonates with various other ways of seeing DI as a socio-medical practice. First, this view lends authority to the clinical framing of DI practices: after all, who else can improve the quality of the outcome other than the clinicians working to improve the success rates for conception and working to reduce the health risks to recipient and baby? Paradoxically, this version of the baby as a successful outcome also then acts to draw a line under the involvement of clinicians (and the semen provider) in any particular case, since it indicates that the goal has been achieved and thus the other participants can now withdraw whilst the recipients embark on a new and essentially different life, as new parents with a young baby. Thus the notion of successful outcome marks a clear boundary between the old life as recipients and the new life as parents. It discourages any detailed consideration of the links between the two and of the processes which led from one social status to the other.

Such a representation therefore helps to constitute the relationships that enable the clinicians to see themselves as 'merely' providing a service to recipients. This then enables clinicians, recipients and to some extent, donors to see the donors as just another part of that service, thus helping to diminish the idea of any connection between donor and baby. Recipients are then able to characterise the semen providers as having little to do with them directly and as being more clearly located in the world of the clinician.

These associations also lead to a tendency to make the person conceived less visible to the wider community who have little direct experience of, or involvement in, DI. As a consequence, they also make the people conceived through DI less visible to each other. Finally, such a representation helps to establish the view that the only successful way to deal with infertility is to have a baby.[13]

The representation of the people who have been conceived as 'children' provides for greater possibilities of seeing them as individuals in their own right and with a future. However, what appears to happen in the context of DI (as in most other contexts) is that the notion of 'the child' produces associations that have less to do with those children's experiences of being children (that is, as active sense-making agents of their own social world) and more to do with the cultural connotations of the child in Western societies (James and Prout 1990). That is, the child is seen as something that is highly valued in its own right, for its special qualities rather than its economic value. In terms of DI, therefore, the expenditure on trying for the child (especially under private medicine) is justified. However, part of that value is derived from the association of childhood with innocence and of being unsullied by adult concerns (Boyden 1990: 185–6). Hence, the view within earlier DI practice that the child could gain nothing from knowing about the connection between his/her conception, the practice of masturbation and the status of illegitimacy. The damage would not only be to his/her identity as a stigmatised individual but also from having to know about sexuality and reproduction as a necessary part of understanding the significance of how s/he was conceived.

This in turn leads quickly to other associations of childhood: for example, that the child's experiences of the social world are best mediated by the adults in his/her life, partly to protect the child from those harsher realities of the world, partly to mediate and interpret those realities when they cannot be avoided. Within the world of DI, these assumptions about children are expressed in the concern for the welfare of the child. Whilst this view is important in encouraging practitioners and recipients to look beyond the successful birth of a healthy baby, it also tends to mean that the child is then seen as essentially passive and silent, as having needs but, as a consequence of those needs, also being vulnerable. As Woodhead (1990) argues, statements about children's needs derive from a view of childhood as a universally similar experience and therefore damaging consequences are threatened if those needs are not met. Certainly this is the way in which the arguments concerning the 'child's' needs for access to genetic information are structured in DI.

There is however a curious feature about those arguments on access to information, in so far as most focus on the idea of the 'child' gaining such information at the age of eighteen, when s/he is going through the transition to adulthood. Thus the assumptions of dependency and passivity of childhood are displaced by an awareness that there may be a more active, independent person emerging who is capable of seeking out such information. Yet, curiously, such awareness tends to stop at this point, where childhood enters into adulthood: there is little sense, in the representations of people conceived by DI, of them as adults beyond the age of eighteen, of what they might look like, of how they might behave, of what they would want, need or like.

Until that is, the DI adults themselves present such accounts. These are important because it is only in such accounts that they obtain a central authorial role: a role in which they are seen to possess agency and status. But, paradoxically, it is these accounts from DI adults themselves that make us fully aware of the representational status of all accounts concerning people conceived by DI. It would be easy to assume that DI adults are the experts and thus the source of the definitive view of 'the person conceived through DI', but even in the few accounts currently available, we find there are variations in personal experience, variations in the interpretation of those experiences and variations in the claims made about what those experiences tell us about DI adults more generally.

Thus in discussing the notion of how the person conceived by DI has been represented by others I am not searching for the one definitive, authoritative account. None of these representations carries any greater authority than the others: they all inform us about the person conceived by DI but, more importantly, they also inform us about the wider relationships around DI as a social practice and of how the person conceived fits within that web.[14] In this chapter we have seen how the person conceived by DI has been and continues to be the product of social relations and social processes. In this way we have seen the making of the 'DI child', both by the process of conception and, more important, by the process of cultural categorisation.

NOTES

1. More general developments in childbirth practices and assisted conception have led Rothman to describe foetuses, babies and children as the 'products of conception' (1985: 188).
2. Previously (Haimes 1992) I have chosen to use the term 'child' to ensure the clarity of which party in the DI process is being referred to, but in so doing I have always put the term in inverted commas to draw attention to its limitations. The term 'offspring' is not a wholly satisfactory alternative since it too tends to emphasise a child-like status and perpetuates the tendency only to see the DI person in relation to his/her parents. Gibson (1991–2: 2) reports a similar difficulty.
3. See Oliver (1990: xiii) for a dissenting view to this however.

4. Whilst this latter point is important from a socio-political point of view, I am more attracted, analytically, by the open-ended aspect of the term.

5. This is a salutary but necessary point to make, otherwise it becomes very easy to slip into referring to those conceived by DI as someone other than 'us', the writers and readers of this material.

6. It is often the case, of course, that even when fairly precise knowledge is held about the numbers affected by an issue, stereotypes about the person concerned and misconceptions about the numbers affected still abound. However, these stereotypes and images can become more powerful when established facts, even about numbers, are missing.

7. Annas felt that the interests of donors and of clinicians, in particular, were allowed to obscure those of the 'children'.

8. For example, in Haimes (1988) I suggest that the claims about the extent of openness in adoption were over-stated. I have also argued (Haimes 1990) that analyses in adoption tend to be reductionist, in their focus on the problems for individuals, rather than on the social context of the practice as a whole.

9. I have argued elsewhere that in the earlier debates over donor anonymity an apparent concern for the child could be seen as an effective protection for the doctors' interests (Haimes 1993).

10. Although, since we do not know how many DI adults know about their conception, we do not know if those who have spoken out are atypical or not.

11. Another group established by adults conceived through donor insemination called HOPE (Help Offspring Pursue Ethics) has also been formed in the United States (Achilles 1995).

12. That these are broad tendencies should be emphasized since it will be apparent from a careful reading of the chapter that representations of the person conceived have to some extent overlapped and have also gone through various changes: for example, from baby/child (in terms of the success of conception) to child/teenager (in terms of the need for 'roots') to child (in terms of welfare needs) to the foetus (in terms of genetic risks) to baby/child (in terms of concerns with development). This emphasizes the point that the history of representations of the person conceived should not be understood as a smooth progression to some favoured understanding, but as a complex set of understandings that have emerged, as different voices and parties have participated in the discussion over DI.

13. Aspects of each of these points are elaborated upon in each of the other chapters in this collection: my aim here is simply to show that these connections exist rather than to spell them out in detail.

14. Hockey and James (1993: 34) quote Geertz's view that persons are perceived 'not baldly . . . as mere unadorned members of the human race, but as representative of certain distinct categories of persons, specific sorts of individuals' (1975: 363). Such representations Geertz says, are 'historically constructed, socially maintained and individually applied' (*ibid*).

REFERENCES

Achilles, R. G. (1986) 'The social meanings of biological ties: a study of participants in artificial insemination by donor'. PhD thesis, Department of Education, University of Toronto.

(1992) *Donor Insemination: an overview.* Royal Commission on New Reproductive Technologies, Ottawa, Canada.

(1995) 'Gamete donation: rationale, design and implementation of an open model'. Unpublished paper.

Adair, V. (1994) 'Issues in the move from anonymity with the use of donor gametes: research evidence'. Paper presented to the Seminar on the Regulation of Assisted Reproductive Technology, Wellington, New Zealand, April 1994.

American Fertility Society (1990) 'New guidelines for the use of semen donor insemination'. *Fertility and Sterility* Supplement 1, 53(3): 1S–12S.

Annas, G. (1980) 'Fathers anonymous: beyond the best interests of the sperm donor'. In A. Milunsky and G. Annas, eds., *Genetics and the Law, II.* New York: Plenum Press.

Artificial Human Insemination: the report of a Commission appointed by His Grace the Archbishop of Canterbury (1948) London: Society for the Propagation of Christian Knowledge.

Barton, M., Walker, K. and Wiesner, B. (1945) 'Artificial insemination'. *British Medical Journal* 1 (Jan.): 40–3.

Benda Kommission des Bundestages (1985) Bundesepublik Deutschland. Bericht der Arbeitsgruppe *Un vitro* Fertilization, Genomanalyse und Gentherapie, Bonn.

Boyden, J. (1990) 'Childhood and the policymakers'. In A. James and A. Prout, eds., *Constructing and reconstructing childhood.* Falmer Press: Basingstoke, pp. 184–215.

Brandon, J. and Warner, J. (1977) 'AID and adoption: some comparisons'. *British Journal of Social Work* 7(3): 335–41.

Brandon, J. (1979) 'Telling the A.I.D. child'. *Adoption and Fostering* 85(1): 13–14.

British Agencies for Adoption and Fostering Medical Group (1984) *AID and After.* London: BAAF.

British Andrology Society (1993) 'Guidelines for the screening of semen donors for donor insemination'. *Human Reproduction* 8(9): 1521–3.

British Medical Association (1973) 'Annual Report of the Council. Appendix V: Report of the Panel on Human Artificial Insemination'. *British Medical Journal* Supplement, April, 2: 3–5 (The 'Peel Report').

Cushan, A.-M., ed. (1984) *Adoption and AID: access to information?* Proceedings of the Conference, Monash University Centre for Human Bioethics, Melbourne, Australia, 1983.

Daniels, K. (1995) 'Policy Directions for Assisted Human Reproduction in New Zealand'. *Journal of Fertility Counselling* 2(1): 14–16.

Department of Health and Social Security (1984) Report of the Committee of Inquiry into Human Fertilization and Embryology ('The Warnock Report'). Cmnd 9314. London: Her Majesty's Stationery Office.

Englert, Y. (1994) 'Artificial insemination of single women and lesbian women with donor semen'. *Human Reproduction* 9(11): 1,969–71.

Feversham Report (1960) Report of the Departmental Committee on Human Artificial Insemination. London: Her Majesty's Stationery Office (Cmnd 1105).

Geertz, C. (1975) *The Interpretation of Culture.* London: Hutchinson.

Gibson, E. (1991–92). 'Artificial insemination by donor: information, communication and regulation', *Journal of Family Law*, 30(1): 1–44.

Golombok, S., Bhanji, F., Rutherford, T. and Winston, R. (1990) 'Psychological development of children of the new reproductive technologies: issues and a pilot study of children conceived by IVF'. *Journal of Reproductive and Infant Psychology* 8(1): 37–43.

Golombok, S., Cook, R., Bish, A. and Murray, C. (1995) 'Families created by the new reproductive technologies: quality of parenting and social and emotional development of the children'. *Child Development* 66(2): 285–98.

Golombok, S. and Tasker, F. (1994) 'Donor insemination for single heterosexual and lesbian women: issues concerning the welfare of the child'. *Human Reproduction* 9(11): 1,972–6.

Haimes, E. (1988) '"Secrecy": what can artificial reproduction learn from adoption?' *International Journal of Law and the Family* 2: 46–61.

(1990) 'Family connections: the management of biological origins in the new reproductive technologies'. PhD thesis, University of Newcastle, UK.

(1992) 'Gamete donation and the social management of genetic origins'. In M. Stacey, ed., *Changing human reproduction*. London: Sage, pp. 119–47.

(1993) 'Do clinicians benefit from gamete donor anonymity?' *Human Reproduction*, 8(9): 1,518–20.

Hockey, J. and James, A. (1993) *Growing up and growing old*. London: Sage.

Holland, J. (1971) 'Adoption and artificial insemination: some social implications'. *Soundings* 50(4): 302–7.

Holmes, H., Hoskins, B. and Gross, M., eds. (1981) *Custom-made child?* Clifton, NJ: Humana Press.

Home Office and Scottish Home Department (1960) Report of the Departmental Committee on Human Artificial Insemination ('The Feversham Report'). Cmnd 1105. London: Her Majesty's Stationery Office.

Human Fertilisation and Embryology Act (1990) London: HMSO.

Humphrey, M. and Humphrey, H. (1986) 'A fresh look at genealogical bewilderment'. *British Journal of Medical Psychology* 59 (Part 2): 133–40.

Iizuka, R., Sawada, Y., Nishina, N. and Ohi, M. (1968) 'The physical and mental development of children born following artificial insemination'. *International Journal of Fertility* 13(1): 24–32.

James, A. and Prout, A., eds. (1990) *Constructing and reconstructing childhood*. Falmer Press: Basingstoke, UK.

Langer, G., Lemberg, E. and Sharf, M. (1969) 'Artificial insemination: a study of 156 cases'. *International Journal of Fertility* 14(3): 232–40.

Leeton, J. and Blackwell, J. (1982) 'A preliminary psychosocial follow-up of parents and their children conceived by artificial insemination by donor'. *Clinical Reproduction and Fertility* 1: 307–10.

Lieberman, B., Matson, P. L. and Hamer, F. (1994) 'The UK Human Fertilisation and Embryology Act, 1990 – how well is it functioning?' *Human Reproduction* 9(9): 1,779–82.

McWhinnie, A. (1982) 'The case for greater openness concerning A.I.D'. Paper presented at the British Agencies for Adoption and Fostering Study Day on AID and Childlessness, November, London, UK.

Morgan, D. and Bernatt, E. (1992) 'The reproductive waltz: the Austrian Act on Procreative Medicine'. *Journal of Social Welfare and Family Law* 5: 420–6.

Novaes, S. (1994) *Les passeurs de gametes*. Nancy: Presses Universitaires de Nancy.

Oliver, M. (1990) *The politics of disablement*. Basingstoke: Macmillan.

Orenstein, P. (1995) 'Looking for a donor to call Dad'. *New York Times Magazine*, 18 June.

Peel Report (1973) 'Report of the Panel on Human Artificial Insemination'. *British Medical Journal*, Supplement, April, 2: 3–5.

Rothman, B. K. (1985) 'The products of conception: the social context of reproductive choices'. *Journal of Medical Ethics* 11: 188–92.

Shenfield, F. (1994a) 'Filiation in assisted reproduction: potential conflicts and legal implications'. *Human Reproduction*, 9(7): 1,348–54.

(1994b) 'Particular requests in donor insemination: comments on the medical duty of care and the welfare of the child'. *Human Reproduction* 9(11): 1,976–7.

Snowden, R. (1990) 'The family and artificial reproduction'. In D. Bromham, M. Daldon and J. Jackson, eds., *Philosophical Ethics in Reproductive Medicine*. Manchester: Manchester University Press.

Snowden, R. and Mitchell, G. D. (1981) *The artificial family*. London: Allen and Unwin.

Snowden, R., Mitchell, G. D. and Snowden, E. (1983) *Artificial reproduction*. London: Allen and Unwin.

Speirs, J. (1988) 'Children's rights to know their identity'. In N. Bruce *et al.*, eds., *Truth and the child*. Edinburgh: Family Care.

Statens Offentliga Utredningar, Sweden (1983) Children Conceived by Artificial Insemination (SOU1983: 42). Stockholm.

Stephenson, P. and Wagner, M. (1991) 'Turkey-baster babies: a view from Europe'. *Milbank Quarterly* 69(1): 45–50.

Turner, C. (nd) The kind of parents all AID children would like to have. Donors' Offspring.

(1982) A baby creation story. Donors' Offspring.

Victoria Government, Australia. Committee to consider the social, ethical and legal issues arising from *in vitro* fertilisation (Chairman: Sir Louis Waller): (a) Interim Report, 1982; (b) Report on Donor Gametes in IVF, 1983; (c) Report on the Disposition of Embryos produced by IVF, 1984. ('Waller Report').

Walters, L. (1987) 'Ethics and the new reproductive technologies: an international review of committee statements'. *Hastings Center Report* Special Supplement, 17(3): 3–9.

Warnock Report. (1984) Report of the Committee of Inquiry into Human Fertilisation and Embryology. Department of Health and Social Security. Cmnd 9314. London: Her Majesty's Stationery Office.

Woodhead, M. (1990) 'Psychology and the cultural construction of children's needs'. In A. James and A. Prout, eds., *Constructing and reconstructing childhood*. Falmer Press: Basingstoke, UK, pp. 60–77.

5   The semen providers

Ken Daniels

Introduction

This chapter has as its focus the men who contribute their semen and who have traditionally been called semen donors. The term 'donor' is unsatisfactory, especially when, as frequently occurs, payment of money is involved. Other terms have been suggested: 'vendor', for a man who sells his semen (Annas 1980), and consignor, for a man who hands over his semen and his rights to it (Blank 1990). In this chapter the term 'provider' is used, as it describes both those who sell and those who gift their semen. While semen providers are being isolated for consideration in this chapter, they can not in fact ever be isolated. Their attitudes and behaviours impact on others and others' attitudes and behaviours impact on them.

Semen providers evoke a variety of reactions. The thankfulness of some recipients is matched with the apprehension of others; different offspring report being thankful, and angry; doctors have concerns about the motivations of some of these men and committees set up to review the whole field reflect views varying from uncertainty, apprehension and disgust, through to the desire to value and applaud those who make this contribution. The fact that little has been known about men who become providers has almost certainly contributed to the variety of views held. Providers have in fact been hidden from public awareness and scrutiny and, as this chapter will show, it is only recently that there has been acknowledgement of their contribution.

The semen provider occupies a unique position in that his task has been to provide a part of himself so that another life can be created, a life that he may not know exists. Even if he does know that this life exists he is not likely to meet that person and will not be able to participate in the upbringing of that person. He is therefore expected to share a part of himself and to receive very little, if any, personal acknowledgement in return. The chapter will consider how money has often been used to provide a form of acknowledgement.

What sorts of men provide semen and why do they do it? What impact do the attitudes and values of the other participants in the process and the com-

munity have on them and to what extent is the semen provider a marginalised person? This chapter is designed to give an overview of the information
that is available on the men who provide semen for other persons, and to
explore the wider implications and meanings of this. It begins by reviewing
how the provider's status has changed from one of obscurity to one of
acknowledgement, and ends with a call for a further move to take place,
from acknowledgement to affirmation and valuing. In between the focus is
on the attempts that have been made to let the provider speak and, emerging from that, what providers are saying about their motivations.
Consideration will be given to the actual and potential impact that involvement has on the provider's family – both the family of which he is a part and
the family to which he has contributed but of which he is not, on a practical basis, a part. The exchange of information between the parties involved
in DI will also be highlighted with specific reference to providers (comple-
menting the contributions of Lasker, Haimes, the Snowdens and Blank in
their chapters) and to the role and power of the medical profession in developing the policy and practice context in which information is either shared
or not (linking with Novaes' chapter). It is hoped that the chapter will also
add to a greater understanding of the meaning of semen provision and providers via the notions of gift dynamics and marginalisation.

It must be noted, however, that while most semen provision occurs as a
response to male infertility and that most providers are anonymous (i.e. not
known to the recipients or the offspring) there are important variations to
this. The first variation is that DI is being increasingly used by lesbian
couples and single women. In such situations physical infertility is replaced
by what might be called social infertility (see Lasker's chapter in this collection). There are also situations where, because of a hereditary condition, a
couple may choose to use DI. The second variation relates to anonymity
and the fact that a recipient, or recipients, may use a known semen provider,
someone who is acceptable to her/them (see chapter by Edwards in this
volume). An extension of the use of the known semen provider is when one
member of a family contributes semen for another member of that family,
e.g. brother for brother. It is important to note that legislation in Sweden
(1985) and Austria (1992) makes it possible for offspring to find out the
identity of the semen provider, and current practice in New Zealand provides for this same possibility. Anonymity, however, remains the dominant
policy.

From obscurity to acknowledgement

A New Zealand gynaecologist told me that in the late 1950s he was sched-
uled to inseminate a woman with donor semen. She and her husband had

travelled 150 km for the appointment, and it was only on their arrival that the doctor remembered he was to have obtained the semen from a friend. In the circumstances he decided to use his own semen. When he reported this to his wife she insisted that he have a vasectomy, which he did. Two years later he saw the couple again when they were asking for further DI in order to provide a sibling for their child. They specifically asked for semen from the same man. The doctor explained that the 'donor' was no longer available. He reported being much relieved that this was the case because he had experienced 'unusual feelings' on seeing the couple and 'his' child sitting in the consulting room.

This example has parallels with the first instance of DI using human semen which was reported in 1909 by Addison Hard. Hard was a student of Dr William Pancoast who, while teaching a class at Jefferson Medical College in 1884, discussed a situation in which the male in a couple was discovered to be azoospermic and the female was found to be perfectly capable of bearing children. The students in this class suggested that a 'hired man' be called in to solve the problem. Dr Pancoast then took a semen sample from the 'best looking member of the class' and inseminated the woman without her consent and while she was anaesthetised. The doctor later reluctantly told the husband and was relieved to find he approved of the doctor's actions but suggested that his wife not be told. In 1909 Addison Hard went to New York 'to shake the hand of the young man' who had resulted from this procedure. It is speculated that this latter action indicates that Addison Hard was perhaps the student from which the semen sample was collected in 1884, and consequently the genetic father of the world's first DI offspring (Gregoire and Mayer 1965). While this frequently quoted case is cited as the first reported instance of DI, Novaes in her chapter in this collection has shown that DI was practised earlier than this in France.

Both of these examples provide very clear evidence for one of the reasons why the 'donors' have traditionally been kept in obscurity. While the two examples occurred some seventy-five years apart, they represent the genesis and continuing thinking about the role and position of the semen provider. Finegold said, 'It is generally agreed that the donor's identity should be veiled in absolute obscurity' (1964: 35), and in 1981 Glezerman wrote that donor semen should be regarded as 'material from an anonymous testis', the donor being actually a 'non-person' (1981: 185). Such a position, if adopted, would represent complete obscurity in that the provider is not even to be considered a person. In those circumstances, the psychosocial factors associated with providing semen do not have to be considered, the focus is on the provision of 'material' and the man is much the same as a machine – a producer of products. Glezerman continues, 'The myth of blood and flesh has to be uprooted and a state of consciousness has to be achieved in which the donor, from the psychologic point of view, does not exist' (1981: 185).

It is important to recognise that part of the obscurity of the semen provider is related to the obscurity that has tended to surround DI in general. In 1989, one author said of DI practice in the United Kingdom that it was 'shrouded in secrecy and silence' (Dewar 1989: 115). Uneasiness about the moral status of a couple who accept gametes from a third party, and the idea that this was akin to adultery, were prevalent in some of the early discussions of DI. The legal implications for offspring, providers and recipient couples were yet further reasons for maintaining the shroud of secrecy (Rowland 1985). Finegold's brief history of DI in the United States demonstrates that greater acceptance and approval of DI was possible once prominent medical professionals became involved in providing the service, illustrating the important and powerful role that the profession has had in the social understanding and acceptability of DI. The origin of keeping semen providers in obscurity can be traced to medical paternalism, which, based on anxiety surrounding the practice itself, led to a desire to protect those who could provide their semen and then walk away. Given that many early semen providers were medical students, there was a sense in which the profession was also protecting itself and its members. With the medical influence came the focus on doctors and their skills and techniques. The provider, in fact, was seen as a means to an end and the control of the process remained firmly in the hands of the doctors.

A review of the literature shows that the beginnings of a recognition of the semen provider as a person with feelings, thoughts and actions, rather than a 'non-person' began in the 1970s. It was at this time that references began to be made to 'donors' in the literature but these references were, at first, brief and made almost in passing. Early scientific DI studies in the 1970s concentrated on medical aspects, for example, the screening of donors and recipients, and on questions of recruitment (Schoysman 1975; Strickler *et al.* 1975; Dixon and Buttram 1976; Joyce 1984), and a British Medical Association Panel on Human Artificial Insemination (1973) made pronouncements on proper procedures and types of donors, approving of the recruitment of medical and dental students. Some papers reported on the outcomes of DI programmes without mentioning the donors except to say that they existed and that no records were available (Dixon and Buttram 1976). The first studies of DI recipients and their experiences make little mention of semen providers (Rubin 1965; Nijs and Rouffa 1975; David and Avidan 1976; Clayton and Kovacs 1980; Rosenkvist 1981; Leeton and Backwell 1982).

In the 1970s, Curie Cohen *et al.* (1979) set out to document DI practice in the United States and, in so doing, described the source of semen providers, and the practices regarding screening and payment. 'Donors' themselves were not, however, contacted, rather the information came from the clinics and sperm banks. During the early 1980s, studies appeared which specifically set out to describe the source of and characteristics of semen providers more systematically, such as Worsnop *et al.* (1982) in Melbourne Australia. However, it is notable that they could not access their subjects directly because they believed that most would be 'sensitive about their anonymity' so instead they asked the people who recruited these men. Recruitment issues and the relative shortage of semen providers were the main focus of this study. More recently, published studies of the medical aspects of donor semen, such as the screening of semen for disease and fertilising ability (McGowan *et al.* 1983; Greenblatt *et al.* 1986; Selva *et al.* 1986; Monteiro *et al.* 1987; Chauhan *et al.* 1988; Barratt *et al.* 1989; Hummel and Talbert 1989; Schroeder-Jenkins and Rothmann 1989; Bordsan and Leonardo 1991; British Andrology Society 1993; American Fertility Society 1993), are still more common than studies of the psychosocial aspects.

It was significant that editorials in the British Medical Journal in 1975 and 1979 suggested that recruiting medical students for semen provision was perhaps not in the best interests of the individuals concerned. This position implies that consideration was being given to the men involved – albeit particular types of men – rather than just their semen. The provider was beginning to be acknowledged. It had taken almost 100 years.

Letting the semen provider speak

As far as can be ascertained, the first study to be reported in the literature resulting from information obtained directly from providers was undertaken by Patrick Huerre in France. He noted that at that time, 'only the donation is mentioned, never the donor' (1980: 462). He wanted to break what he described as 'a heavy silence, only occasionally replaced by personal fantasising [that] hangs over this subject' (1980: 461). Huerre was able to speak to all forty-five providers who were involved in one clinic. There seemed to be no reluctance on the part of these men, some accompanied by their wives to take part in the study. In this study it is possible to hear the semen providers' voices for the first time.

The study reported by Daniels (1987) required the approval of five different ethical committees. The intention was to ask respondents if, having completed the postal questionnaire, they would be prepared to take part in a follow-up personal interview. If they agreed to this, they were to supply their names and addresses so that direct contact could be made, rather than through the five clinics involved. Two ethics committees refused permission for this opportunity to be given to respondents, on the basis that it would allow the researcher to identify them, and this would breach the promised anonymity. It has to be emphasised that what was proposed meant that the semen providers themselves would make that decision. It is significant that in the three clinics where semen providers were given this opportunity, twenty out of twenty-three gave their names and addresses. This suggests that semen providers did want to speak for themselves and did want to take part in the study to share their views, but ethical committee paternalism in two situations would not allow this.

Extremely high response rates to semen provider surveys (Daniels 1987, 1989; Daniels *et al.* 1996) have been reported. This would point to a desire on the part of the semen providers to be able to speak. Robyn Rowland, in an Australian study, involving a self-completion questionnaire, reported that 'more donors requested interviews than could be seen, indicating the need to have a person available for discussion with them' (1983: 257). Rowland believed that counselling for semen providers was essential so that issues could be discussed and informed consent given. The issue of counselling for semen providers, or perhaps more appropriately, meeting the psychosocial needs of semen providers, will be returned to in the conclusion to this chapter.

In the fifteen years since Huerre reported the results of his study, twenty-two further papers, reports or conference presentations which have reported the views of semen providers have been located. Sixteen of these have appeared in journals or books, and cover the countries of France, United Kingdom, the United States, Canada, Australia, New Zealand, Denmark, Belgium and Czechoslovakia. The discipline of the authors seems to have changed in that earlier studies were in the main carried out by medical doctors, whereas in the latter part of the fifteen-year period there has been an increasing number of social scientists involved. This confirms the growing acceptance of the need to study the psychosocial factors associated with semen provision and providers, as well as the 'opening up' of the area of study to non-medical personnel. What has been most exciting from the point of view of a holistic approach to the subject, has been the development of a team approach to this field of study; these teams often including medical, scientific, and social science personnel.

The results of studies in which semen providers have been given the opportunity to speak, are now reviewed. The particular focus is the motivations of semen providers for involvement, their family relationships, and their views concerning the sharing of information. These three areas are being highlighted because they are of considerable psychosocial importance and interest and lie at the heart of the social and psychological dimension of family creation by means of DI.

The motivations of semen providers

What motivates some men to provide their semen for others? The answer to this question is dependent on which semen providers are giving their reasons – younger men who are predominantly students tend to have quite different reasons than older men who are married or in permanent relationships and have children within that family grouping. Further analysis of the semen provider studies shows that the clinic, programme or doctor who has recruited the semen provider is likely to have an influence on the provider's reported motivations.

The following two quotations illustrate the reasons cited most frequently in studies for becoming a semen provider.

I love children so much and I have so many nice times with my children, and we [provider and his wife] wanted to give other people the same happiness and so it was important for us and we try to help other people. (from Daniels *et al.* 1996: 747)

I was totally penniless and I needed a small regular income with which to continue job search. The alternative was to become an accountant! More interesting jobs take time to get. I don't really mind about contributing to conception (although perhaps I would prefer not to) especially if it is to help infertile fathers. (Daniels *et al.* (1996: 747)

The first of these statements talks of the desire to give other people happiness, along with a desire to help people. The second talks of money as being the main motivation, although the semen provider did not 'mind' contributing to a conception if it was to help infertile fathers. Altruistic reasons or financial reward, or some combination of the two is what most semen providers report as being their reasons for becoming involved. Three other reasons appear in some of the studies; the desire to test one's own fertility; a desire to procreate; and sexual satisfaction.

The type of provider recruited along with his motivations are influenced by whether or not there is a policy of payment for semen. Novaes has said, 'The fact that . . . the donor is almost always remunerated indicates that semen donation is defined in advance as a commercial transaction, when in fact its meaning for the donor – and for society – may be totally different' (1989: 643). It is for this reason that the policies adopted by clinics and programmes are so central to the recruitment of semen providers. A recent paper by Daniels and Lewis (1996a) has reviewed the issue of the commercialisation of semen, and in so doing points to the role occupied by health professionals – namely that of brokers or mediators. DI practitioners are, in the commercial model, both buyers and sellers of semen, buying from the provider and then on-selling frozen 'straws' to clients, usually with a price mark-up to allow for the costs of recruitment, screening and payment of providers, testing and storage and possibly (but certainly not in all cases) a profit margin. Sperm banks represent a form of semen provision that is one step removed from this in that another broker is involved (see Lasker's chapter in this volume). In the non-commercial model, the health professional acts as a broker, but without payment being made to the provider. Yet another model may operate when 'personal' or 'known' providers are used and the health professional then fulfils a mediating role.

The advantages of the commercialised model have been advocated by health professionals for two reasons. First, it assists in recruiting providers (but only if potential semen providers are in need of money) and, second, payment may be seen to finalise the transaction and remove the idea that providers are owed anything further, such as information about outcomes, counselling or social recognition. It is interesting to note that the UK Warnock Committee (1984) recommended that reimbursement be available to 'donors' under conditions of licence. The Human Fertilisation and Embryology Authority, in its 1996 Annual Report, says that it has now decided to phase out payments to donors and benefits in kind, apart from the reimbursement of reasonable direct expenses. A working group has been established to consider how to withdraw payments and the date from which payments will cease completely (HFEA 1996). The American Fertility Society (1986) recommended donors be remunerated, but that they should not receive so much that monetary concerns become the primary motivation for donating. As the Glover Report to the European Commission (1989) noted, the French CECOS (Centre d'Etude et Conservation du Sperme) Federation clinics do not pay or reimburse donors' expenses. The report observed that, in general, while some men may provide sperm for money, payment may give other men a 'reason' to donate which allows them to avoid examining their real motives. On the other hand, the Report noted that payment takes away the chance for these men to do something purely for others. Ultimately, the Glover Report (1989) recommended policies to promote 'altruistic' donating, payment only to be used as a last resort to make up provider shortfalls. In Canada, the recent Royal Commission on New Reproductive Technologies (1993) recommended that semen providers be 'reimbursed', but not more than the current amount of $75, as more may constitute a financial incentive. A recent Bill introduced by the Canadian Government (Bill C-47) bans not only payment for the gametes, but also bans the reimbursement of expenses

Turning from the issue of payment as a given to how semen providers themselves describe their motivations, Table 5.1 presents data obtained from twenty studies undertaken in different parts of the world.

While it is not possible to drawn firm conclusions from the results of these studies, some trends seem to be clearly evident. The first such

Table 5.1. *Studies of the motivation of semen providers*

Author/s	Year	Country	Age	Occupation	Marital status	Children of own	Motivation	Monetary consideration
Huerre	1980	France	Mean age=32	'Socially & professionally predominantly above-average'	All married or in steady relationship	Not reported	Primarily to help	Not paid
Kovacs *et al.*	1983	Australia	64%=18–20 36%=25–40	Not reported	84%=single 16%=married	8%	92% to help 88% money 24% to father children 20% pass on genes	Paid 64% would still provide without payment 36% would still provide but would be less motivated
Nicholas & Tyler	1983	Australia	Range 22–50 Majority in late 20s– early 30s	24% management 18% skilled manual 18% unskilled manual 16% professional 14% clerical 10% student	54% married or in stable relationship	44%	68% to help 8% money 24% other reasons	'Most' would provide without payment 40% thought there should be a payment
Rowland	1983	Australia	Median 31 Range 19–49	Not reported but: 9% upper class 58% middle class 30% student	58% married or living together 24% single 8% separated/divorced	35%	61% to help 24% money 7% knew infertile couple	Paid 57% would provide without payment 39% would not provide without payment 83% thought there should be payment

Study	Country	Age	Occupation	Marital status	Not reported	Motivation	Payment
Handelsmann et al.	1985	Australia	Not reported	Not reported	52% married	Not reported	91% to help 43% evaluate fertility 49% procreate 11% money	Paid Money important to 16% Single men more interested in money
Nijs & Rouffa	1986	Belgium	Mean (unmarried)=24 Mean (married)=29	74% student 26% professional	85% single 11% married 4% divorced	11%	Predominately to help	Paid Money a secondary motivation, but did provide impetus to provide
Paul & Durna	1987	Australia	17%=18–29 68%=30–40 12%=above 40	64% professional	62% married	56%	100% to help 12% evaluate fertility 0% finance 26% other – mainly genetic continuity	Not paid and finance not an issue
Daniels	1987	New Zealand	Median 31 Range 22–52	62% professional 14% sales/service 16% student	65% married/living together 27% single 8% previously married	62%	91% to help 24% money 14% evaluate fertility	28% expected payment 51% received payment 43% disapproved of payment 60% would provide without payment
Daniels	1989	Australia	Median 34.5 Range 19–42	63% professional 14% sales/service 14% student 9% production	36% married/living together 50% single 14% previously married	50%	91% to help 32% money 36% evaluate fertility	86% received payment, but only 41% expected it 50% money important 50% money not important 59% would provide without payment

Table 5.1 (*cont.*)

Author/s	Year	Country	Age	Occupation	Marital status	Children of own	Motivation	Monetary consideration
Sauer *et al.*	1989	USA	Range = 21–30	100% physician, house staff or students	75% single 25% married	Not reported	62% money	Paid and expected to be paid Majority would not provide without payment
Fidell & Marik	1989	USA	Mean = 28 Range = 19–48	50% students, remainder mainly professionals	64% single 21% married 15% previously married	23%	74% money 15% to help 8% procreate	Money primary motivation but 41% would provide without payment
Mahlstedt & Probasco	1991	USA	Median 24	82% students	57% single	Not reported	67% altruism = a reason 63% financial gain = a reason	Not reported
Blood	1992	Australia	29% = 18–25 50% = 26–35 21% = 36–45	'Good variety' 20% students	48% married 44% single 8% divorced	44%	100% to help 29% evaluate fertility 21% financial reasons 18% father a child	All paid but 95% prepared to provide if no remuneration
Chapman & Crittenden	1992	Australia	Median 34 Range 19–53	Not reported	36% married 27% steady relationship 27% single	Not reported	83% altruism 7% money	52% approved of payments

Study	Year	Country	Age	Occupation	Marital status		Motivation	Comments
Schover et al.	1992	USA	Mean 28.5	65% student 18% professional	59% single 35% married 6% divorced	30%	71% money 29% to help	Unlikely to provide without payment as this is the primary motivation
Pedersen et al.	1994	Denmark	Mean 26.9 Range=21–35	'Almost all university students'	Not reported	Not reported	32% financial 8% altruism 60% combination of above	'Finance found to be more or less important to 92%' Not paid, but provided with travelling expenses.
Lui et al.	1995	UK	Range=18–34 77% under 22	'Majority were students'	Not reported	Not reported	81% to help 69% financial reward	69% would not provide semen without payment 45% thought donors should be paid more
Cook & Golombok	1995	UK	Mean 24 71% 21 or over 37% 25 or over	65% students 11% unemployed 26% paid employment	81% single 15% married/ living together	15%	70% money very or moderately important 79% helping very or moderately important	99% believed they should be paid at least at current rate. 62% would not provide without payment 'A significantly greater proportion of older donors than younger donors would donate without payment.'

Table 5.1 (*cont.*)

Author/s	Year	Country	Age	Occupation	Marital status	Children of own	Motivation	Monetary consideration
Daniels *et al.* Clinic A	1996	UK	Median 41 Mean 40 Range 31–51	53% professional 35% clerical, trades/ self employed	76% married 18% previously married 9% single	94%	100% to help 6% to procreate 6% evaluate fertility	82% shouldn't be paid 18% should be paid 29% should be given expenses
Clinic B			Median 24 Mean 27 Range 20–40	45% student 36% professional	91% single 9% married	9%	82% money 63% to help 27% evaluate fertility 9% procreate	73% should be paid 63% should be given expenses
Daniels *et al.*	1997	Sweden	Median 37 Range 21–53	53% professional 23% services/sales 12% students	35% married 35% single 28% living together	67%	88% to help 30% money 23% evaluate fertility	63% approved of payments 23% disapproved of payments

trend/observation is that age, marital status, children, occupation and reasons for providing semen are interlinked. Cook and Golombok (1995) made the observation that studies seem to reveal that financial motivation is more likely to be associated with 'donor' populations dominated by students and Barratt (1993) has pointed out that students account for about 75 per cent of semen providers in the United Kingdom. A second observation is that the motivation for becoming a semen provider seems to vary between clinics and this is very clear in the case of the Daniels *et al.* study (1996). The two clinics differed in their recruitment policies and this is reflected in the motivations of the recruits.

It is also possible to note a trend which shows that the commercial model seems to be less important in Australia and New Zealand than it is, for example, in the United States. It could be very easy to conclude that this represents a cultural difference, similar to that noted by Titmuss (1970) in relation to the provision of blood. However, it seems more likely that the differences relate to recruitment demands and the policies of different clinics: a difference that can be summarised as being related to the convenience of recruiting students and to the avoidance of having to deal with the psychosocial aspects of semen provision and their importance in gift dynamics and kin relationships. In a recent review of the gifting and selling of semen by Daniels and Lewis (1996a), it was concluded that the medical construction of semen provision as a commercial transaction may have driven away some potential donors.

Semen providers and their families

The semen provider is actually, or potentially, a part of two family groupings. If he is married or in a continuing relationship, and he and his partner have children, then this is regarded as his family. He and his partner are linked to their children genetically, legally, psychosocially and culturally. As a semen provider he has genetic links to another child (or children), who is going to be brought up as part of a family. His psychosocial involvement with this child and her/his parents is likely to be very limited, in fact probably in most situations non-existent. The use of the word 'family' presents difficulties in this connection, in that family is normally accepted as being based on kin relationships. How then do we describe the situations where a semen provider has provided a genetic contribution to a child, but has no links apart from this? (see chapter by Edwards in this collection) At the heart of this issue lies the importance that is placed on biological and social notions of parenthood (Stacey 1992; Strathern 1992). Purdie *et al.* have aptly pointed out that 'a man is a sperm donor for only a short time; after that he is a man with children in someone else's family' (1994: 1358).

As long as the emphasis was on the semen only, with providers seen as a means to an end and as having no interest in the outcomes of their contributions, these issues could be avoided. Schoysman sums up this position when he says:

Not only do we believe that the donor should never know who the recipients are but we do not even tell him whether there was a success or not. To tell a donor, for instance, that a boy has been obtained thanks to his contribution may be accepted without comment at the time . . . but if in the future something happens to his own children, it is very likely that later in life he will be troubled by the fact that somewhere there is another child of his alive. So the donor is given no information. He contributes by giving a semen sample but there is no reason whatsoever that he should know the result. (1975: 35)

Or as Johnston says:

Apart from the usual medical grounds for rejection an occasional person will not be considered if he seems unusually interested in the progeny that may be produced from his semen. The absolute anonymity of the donor is considered essential in this country and all donors must be prepared to donate semen without any follow-up information on its use or results. (1980: 14–15)

Semen providers themselves do not see the issue in this way. This has been demonstrated in several studies. In studies by Daniels (1987, 1989) 38 per cent and 96 per cent were very interested or interested in knowing the outcome of their contributions and in another study in Sweden by Daniels, 60 per cent were interested (under editorial review). Purdie *et al.* (1992) found that 80 per cent wanted to know if children were conceived; Mahlstedt and Probasco (1991) found that 41 per cent wanted to know if pregnancies had occurred; Fidell and Marik (1989) found that 69 per cent wanted to know if there were any children and many of these would have liked a picture; Handelsmann *et al.* (1985) found that 63 per cent wanted to know if pregnancies had occurred; Kovacs *et al.* (1983) found that 59 per cent wanted to know if a birth or births had occurred; Rowland (1983) found that 81 per cent wanted to know if children were born; Sauer *et al.* (1989) found that 79 per cent were interested in knowing the outcomes of their donations; and Chapman and Crittenden (1992) found that 27 per cent reported they did not like having no information about progeny. From this review it is clear that the majority of semen providers in many different countries in the world, and operating within different clinic policies, wish to have information concerning the outcomes of their contributions.

Other indications of the provider feeling a link or bond between himself and his offspring are reflected in the fact that 72 per cent of one group of providers wanted to leave a message for their offspring (Mahlstedt and Probasco 1991); 36 per cent in another group would like to meet the offspring (Sauer *et al.* 1989); many would like a photograph and 21 per cent of one group felt some sense of responsibility towards the offspring (Fidell and Marik 1989). In a study undertaken by Daniels, Ericsson and Burn, 74 per cent think about the offspring created by DI (1996) and by Daniels, 72 per cent sometimes think about the offspring (1989); and 68 per cent think about the possible DI offspring (1987).

Although some health professionals have denied provider interest, or tried to 'select out' those who expressed interest, it is clear that the interest is there. Perhaps it is because of the lack of responsiveness to the psycho-social needs of semen providers, especially in areas such as having offspring that they feel some link or bond with, that a number of writers are starting to report that some providers are expressing regrets about having been involved in earlier years (Baran and Pannor 1989; Brandon and Warner 1977; Curson and Daniels, under editorial review).

The semen provider's relationships with his family also need to be con-sidered. An analysis of the various studies indicates that the majority of semen providers have shared with their partners and close friends the fact that they have provided semen for DI. This is not surprising given the importance of the decision, but it is also interesting that there are still many providers who have not told partners, or will not tell future partners if they are currently single. Some early practitioners, and perhaps some modern ones, see the involvement of the partner as another source of potential complications. Finegold wrote in 1964: 'We prefer single men . . . Because most physicians who choose married donors insist that the donor's wife be informed, we feel this adds another person who can provide further prob-lems to the many uncertainties of A.I.' (1964: 36). Today, in the United Kingdom, the HFEA's Code of Practice (1993) recommends but does not require that the semen provider's partner's consent be obtained by the pro-gramme prior to any semen donations.

The possibility of 'known' or 'personal' providers is also of some inter-est. In this situation, an infertile couple (usually) will arrange for someone they know, who may be a relative or a friend, to provide the semen. The Glover Report (1989) notes that some families prefer known 'donors', and explores the reasons for this. The Report sees no general presumption for or against related 'donors', though it does argue that children should not be deceived about relationships. The use of known providers highlights the fact that all the parties are members of one family, if the provider is a rela-tive.

The exchange of information

Arising out of a consideration of the semen provider and his part (actual or potential) in two families, is the question of the exchange of information between those involved. What knowledge, if any, is the DI offspring to have? Can she/he meet the semen provider at some stage in the future? What does the semen provider know about the recipient/s and vice versa? This area has tended to be treated with a great deal of anxiety and uncertainty. The literature has traditionally used words such as secrecy, anonymity, confidentiality, privacy and openness (Snowden *et al.* 1983) to characterise the nature of the relationships between the parties, as well as the sharing of information between them. Some quotations from Finegold illustrate this point well:

The sperm is obtained at seven in the morning and is brought by the student to our office by half past eight . . . Our A.I.D. patients arrive between nine and nine-thirty. Naturally, the donors and the recipients never meet. (1964: 36)

Today all sterologists insist that the donors remain anonymous. (1964: 33)

One of the great values of A.I. is its secrecy. Couples who will expose to friends and relatives the fact that their child is not the biological issue of the husband must not be invited to partake of the procedure. (1964: 32)

In addition, Finegold outlined the lengths to which he and other practitioners went to ensure the identity of semen providers could never be later ascertained, for example, pooling the semen of several providers and never listing the names of providers on patients' files. What is clear from the above quotations and from the general thrust of the literature advocating secrecy is that there is an extremely strong element of protectionism, and in some situations medical paternalism, involved (Daniels 1995). All of the parties involved in DI, the recipients, the semen provider, the offspring, and the health professionals, have been cited by different authors as being in need of protection from the truth, or information associated with the truth (Daniels and Taylor 1993). While health professionals, and in particular, medical practitioners, have played a major part in advocating that there should be no, or very limited, exchange of information between the parties, the recipient couple or individual may also decide to withhold information from their offspring, relatives or friends, believing this to be in their best interests. As a respondent in Snowden, Mitchell and Snowden's study said when asked about telling her children, 'Never, never. I think it would be awful . . . it would be the same as saying to them "he's not really your daddy". No way – I just couldn't' (1983: 118).

The arguments in support of secrecy and openness in DI have been reviewed by Daniels and Taylor (1993) and also by Lasker, the Snowdens, Haimes and Novaes in this collection. What is of significance for this discussion is that it has been argued that if anonymity was not guaranteed for semen providers, then they would not be prepared to come forward (Schoysman 1975; Johnston 1980; Beck 1984; Joyce 1984; Braude *et al.* 1990). Two sources of information present major challenges to this position. The first relates to developments in Sweden following the introduction of legislation making it mandatory for semen providers to record identifying information for their offspring, and for this information to be available to the offspring. Back and Snowden (1988), and Daniels (1994) have pointed out that following the passing of the legislation there was a decline in the number of available semen providers, but that this was short lived. Daniels (1994) and Daniels and Lalos, (1995) comment on the medical profession's involvement in this legislative change, pointing out that the majority of them were opposed to the legislation and that this opposition continued after the legislation was enacted. Studies of semen providers in Sweden indicate that the lack of anonymity is not an impediment to involvement as a semen provider.

The second source of information is that which is available from studies in which the semen providers are given an opportunity to express their views on the matter. In Australia: Nicholas and Tyler (1983) report that 56 per cent of men in their study supported the idea of a national register of names and addresses of providers and recipients; Rowland (1983) found that over half (60 per cent) of the respondents would not mind a meeting with the child at the age of eighteen years; Paul and Durna (1987) found that 59 per cent would agree to their DI offspring making personal contact; and Daniels (1989) found that 68 per cent would not mind if identifying information were given to DI offspring at age eighteen such as would enable them to trace the provider and 73 per cent would still provide semen if they could be traced. Condon and Harrison (1992) reported that 52 per cent of semen providers in their study would be less willing to provide semen without anonymity, and 29 per cent would definitely not provide, reflecting a strong opposition to information about them being given to recipients of their semen at the birth or later. However, 29 per cent would like to meet the child at eighteen. Blood (1992) reported that 37 per cent of respondents in her study wanted complete anonymity but that 59 per cent did not, and that 45 per cent said that if contacted later they would agree to their name being released.

In New Zealand, Daniels (1987) found that one quarter of the semen providers questioned would still be prepared to provide even if offspring were later able to trace them. A more recent study in New Zealand (Purdie *et al.* 1992) found that 68 per cent of the men questioned were agreeable to their identity being made available to their DI offspring when s/he had reached maturity. It should be noted that DI practice in New Zealand, in a matter of a decade, has changed quite dramatically in favour of greater information sharing especially in regard to allowing the resulting 'children' eventually to learn about their provider if they wish. A recent Ministerial Committee (1994) found that, in contrast to the former aura of secrecy which had surrounded gamete provision most, although not all, programmes now have a policy of advising providers and recipients to adopt openness about genetic origins and many providers of services now recruit identifiable providers, i.e. those willing to be identified to offspring in the future. There is little doubt that the cultural influences of the Maori, with their emphasis on knowing one's *whakapapa* (genealogy) was important in this movement towards openness. (For a discussion of this issue, see Ministerial Committee Report 1994; Daniels and Lewis 1996b and Fisher and Peek 1994.) One clinic in New Zealand has even gone as far as no longer offering providers the option of remaining anonymous (Fisher and Peek 1994). The Ministerial Committee gave official support to this movement towards greater openness by recommending that systems be set in place to ensure that DI offspring would ultimately have access to the identity of their semen provider.

In a recent comparative study of semen providers from two UK clinics (Daniels *et al.* 1996) contrasting responses to the question of anonymity and tracing were found. Respondents from both clinics had generally positive attitudes towards the storage of identifying information in a Central Register. However, 41 per cent of men from one clinic (mainly older married men with children of their own, and with primarily altruistic motives) were willing to continue providing if resulting offspring could eventually learn their identity, and a further 18 per cent were unsure. Asked how they would feel if they were traced by offspring, 35 per cent of this group said they would be very unhappy about this, but 53 per cent said they would not mind or would welcome this event. Forty-one per cent thought that the offspring should be able to learn the identity of the semen provider when they reach the age of eighteen. In contrast, men in the second group (in the main unmarried senior students or young professionals whose primary motivation was often financial but who were also pleased to be able to help the infertile) were generally unwilling to continue providing semen under these circumstances (63 per cent), with only 18 per cent being willing; 73 per cent said they would be unhappy if they were traced; and 63 per cent thought that adult offspring should not be able to learn the semen provider's identity.

The above evidence presents significant challenges to the traditionally held view that anonymity was essential to ensure the recruitment of semen providers. This traditional view is perhaps best captured in a 1984 editorial in Fertility and Sterility (Beck 1984) where it was said that, 'we have a definite responsibility to the donor which would be jeopardised with disclosure of the process. There will be no more A.I.D anywhere if the donor thinks his privacy and his protection are threatened' (p. 194).

It is also interesting to note that the Glover Report said that 'there may be more dignity for the donor in a system of openness rather than anonymity' (1989: 36). The authors of the Report prefer a presumption in favour of openness with protection for all parties, which in the case of semen providers would mean protection from claims of paternity. The Asche Committee (1985) in Australia recommended that offspring under eighteen should be given access to non-identifying information, and those eighteen or over should have access to identifying information. The development of registers of information (for example, in the United Kingdom under the auspices of the HFEA) demonstrates a recognition of the need to collect and maintain information. Provisions are usually made for access to that information, but these are very limited.

Changes in the approach to the exchange of information between the involved parties are occurring. Registers and non-identifying information represent a significant shift from the absolute secrecy of earlier years. The developments in New Zealand, Sweden, and Austria, point to how much this is currently in the process of change. A government bill recently introduced in the Victorian State Parliament in Australia (1995) also provides for offspring when eighteen years of age or older to obtain information from which the semen provider will or may be identified. In the conclusion of a paper reporting a UK study (Daniels *et al.* 1997) it is suggested that the absolutist position relating to information that has been adopted in the United Kingdom might in fact be modified to meet the wishes of the semen providers and, in the future, the needs of the offspring. It is argued that, while some men who provide their semen do not favour DI offspring having an automatic right to trace them, some are willing to contemplate being identifiable in the future if the process were handled through an intermediary, and if they had the power to veto the process. If details on the HFEA's register were kept up to date, then semen providers could be contacted by the Authority on behalf of offspring in the future, and these men could choose at that point in time whether to identify themselves. It is hypothesised that many more would at least consider greater information sharing if it were presented in this way, and some offspring could benefit from voluntary openness if the regulations could accommodate this. At present, the legislation makes it clear that, barring exceptional cases (such as where disabled offspring wish to sue the semen provider for neglecting to reveal a family history of an inherited disease), the identity of semen providers will not be divulged. Perhaps it is time for official policies regarding the use of third party gametes to reflect a less paternalistic attitude.

Towards an understanding of the semen provider and his actions

Semen provision, as in DI, has presented major challenges to the way in which fatherhood, family and kin relationships are thought of. This book attempts to provide some understanding of and insights into the nature of those challenges and the ways in which they can be responded to. The semen provider presents perhaps the most powerful challenges, and it is argued that because of these challenges there has been a tendency to ignore these men. When they have been acknowledged, the predominant theme has been one of protecting them from detailed scrutiny, and as a result, depriving them of support and being valued. As the chapter indicates, however, when semen providers are given the opportunity to speak for themselves, a different and often confusing picture begins to emerge. The chapter has highlighted some of the reasons for this, and in particular the significant role that the medical profession has played in creating the 'culture' that has surrounded the men who provide their semen.

Perhaps the central issue relating to an understanding of the semen provider is whether he is to be seen as a machine that produces semen for other people's use, or a man who is giving a part of himself so that a new life can be created, a life that will be genetically linked to him forever. It is this latter thinking that led Baran and Pannor to refer to the semen provider as 'the genetic donor father', and to make the following recommendation:

[He] must accept the lifelong responsibility he bears as a genetic parent of a donor offspring. Providing sperm for insemination carried with it the acceptance of the fact that the donor is half of the biological inheritance of the child produced. That acceptance in turn carries with it a solemn obligation to fulfil the responsibilities inherent to being a genetic donor father. (1989: 170)

The studies reviewed in this chapter point increasingly to a large number of semen providers not only seeing themselves as making an important contribution to other people's lives for altruistic reasons, but also wanting to be seen in this way by others. These are men for whom the psychosocial aspects of DI are important. There is a need to both acknowledge and respond to these men.

The semen provider gives a core part of himself through his semen; it could be said that he is in effect giving himself. In this respect he is very different from a blood donor or an organ donor. These people certainly provide a part of themselves, but that part is of a different order in that it enables another life to be maintained, rather than created. It is also different in that it does not represent a giving of oneself (but rather a part) as is the case in semen provision. Such provision, especially when it is given as a gift, goes to the heart of the meaning and significance of fatherhood and life. In a review of the gifting and selling of semen, already referred to (Daniels and Lewis 1996a), it is argued that theory relating to 'gift dynamics' is highly relevant to the understanding of semen provision. Drawing on the work of Marcel Mauss (1954) and its more recent application in the area of biomedicine by Murray (1987), Novaes (1989), and Fox and Swazey (1978: 1992), it is clear that the 'culture' of gift giving is a very important part of social interaction between people involved in DI. Mauss (1954) wrote that the receiving of a gift creates a powerful obligation in the receiver to reciprocate: reciprocity is the essence of the gift. The more significant the gift, the more powerful the obligation to reciprocate. In cases where an equivalent or similar gift cannot be returned, a 'tyranny of the gift' is possible whereby recipients feel burdened by indebtedness and may become vulnerable to being controlled or manipulated in some way by their 'creditor'. It has been noted that some individuals or groups make gifts specifically with the purpose of controlling the behaviour of others (Murray 1987; Bell and Newby 1976).

Some gifts made possible by modern medicine are inherently non-reciprocal. It was because of the disturbing dynamics that surrounded some early organ transplants that medical teams gradually set in place procedures for anticipating and preventing the tyranny of the gift (Fox and Swazey 1992). For example, a potential donor (e.g. sibling or other family member) might be told that his/her tissue was not compatible with the would-be recipient's when in fact the real grounds for exclusion were psychological: the recipient may have privately expressed apprehension about owing a particular person such a great debt or apprehension about that person taking a serious risk on their behalf. On other occasions, transplant teams observed the family dynamics operating and made a decision based on the likely outcome of introducing powerful gift-dynamics into an already strained situation. It is interesting that Fox and Swazey believe that 'The giving and receiving of a gift of enormous value . . . is the most significant meaning of human organ transplantation' (1978: 5). Furthermore, they note that this gift 'takes place within a complex network of personal relationships that extends to families, the physicians, and all the members of the medical team who are involved in the operation' (1978: 5). This psychosocial perspective of biomedical gifts can be applied to semen provision.

Through the involvement of health professionals as intermediaries, current DI practice seeks to avoid a tyranny of the gift. It creates a safe space in which something of enormous significance (the potential to have a child) can be received from another person without threat to the newly formed family. However, this is achieved by denying the existence of the gift in two ways: by making the gift not a gift, i.e. by paying for it, and through a tight control of information, i.e. anonymity and secrecy. This book, with its focus on the social science dimensions, challenges the view that has dominated DI, namely that commercialisation, depersonalisation of the semen provider and a 'black out' of information exchange between the parties is appropriate. Novaes sums this up well when she asks the question:

Are donors sources of biologic material or partners in a procreative procedure? . . .
Keeping the donor at a distance to avoid the kinship issues latent in such transactions seems to be the main preoccupation of most donor policies and the principal justification for the existence of intermediaries. We have seen how certain uses of compensation, anonymity and screening can allow the donor – and the intermediary – to circumvent questions of meaning. (1989: 654–5)

Another perspective on the semen provider can be provided via the notion of marginalisation. Infertile people, lesbian couples and single women who are the starting point for most DI treatments, usually describe themselves and their experiences in terms which identify them as marginalised people: they are unable to meet the 'norms' of society. Donor insemination as a procedure has tended to have a marginalised status, for the reasons outlined earlier in this chapter. The early medical practitioners who offered DI did so in a way which suggests they felt that their activities in this respect were marginalised, and that they in turn would be marginalised if there was public knowledge of their involvement in providing this service. Finally, the semen provider has been treated as a marginalised person by the medical profession and clinic staff. The emphasis on secrecy and anonymity has confirmed or reinforced this marginal status. The move to acknowledge the semen providers and to allow them to speak has provided the opportunity to question this status.

The marginal status of the semen provider and semen provision in general is reinforced by news media headlines such as 'Four Charged in Illegal Sperm Bank' (*New York Times*, 27 April 1992); 'Mother Accuses Sperm Bank of a Mix-up' (*New York Times*, 9 March 1990); 'Betrayal of Trust. A fertility doctor is accused of secretly fathering as many as 75 children' (*People*, 3 September 1992). It can be argued that such events are more likely to occur when procedures and people are marginalised and not open to public scrutiny and accountability.

Another example of the marginalised status of DI and its participants is the lack of adequate provision for the collection of semen in some clinics. For men to have to use a toilet cubicle to masturbate and produce their semen sample is not according them a status or recognition that is in keeping with them making a gift of life. On the other hand, if the goal is to depersonalise the process as much as possible and to treat men as semen producing machines, then the use of a toilet may be seen as appropriate.

According the semen provider an appropriate level of recognition requires acknowledging the psychosocial factors involved. The Warnock Committee (1984), the Canadian Royal Commission on New Reproductive Technologies (1994) and the Demack Committee in Queensland, Australia (1984) all argued for counselling to be made available to semen providers. The Demack Report stressed the need to inform semen providers about the current debates concerning the right to identifying information. The word counselling, when used in relation to infertility and assisted reproduction, is seen to have several meanings (Daniels 1993). The notions of information counselling, support counselling and therapeutic counselling need to be clearly understood and distinguished. If the word counselling is to be used in relation to semen providers, then the emphasis is almost certainly going to be on the information, implications and support dimensions. Mahlstedt and Greenfeld (1989) have argued in relation to couples seeking assisted reproductive interventions, that the emphasis should be on patient preparation rather than counselling. This would seem to be a very useful notion to apply to meeting the psychosocial issues/needs that arise from becoming a provider of semen. The use of the word counselling, especially with its traditional therapeutic emphasis, may only serve to further marginalise these men.

Conclusion

This chapter has acknowledged that semen providers evoke a variety of reactions, many of these being based on issues to do with what motivates these men to become involved. While semen providers remained shadowy figures, confined to obscurity, the fears and anxieties about their motivations were considerable. With the growing acknowledgement of the semen provider's task and contribution, there has come the opportunity to speak to them and to hear directly what motivates them. The resultant picture has challenged the viewpoints previously expressed on their behalf by doctors and health professionals. Committees of inquiry have begun not only to acknowledge the semen provider, but to make recommendations concerning the ways in which they should be responded to. At the least, the information that is now available enables some of the earlier views, perhaps better described as myths, to be challenged. At best, the information leads to the acknowledgement of many semen providers as men who are concerned for and interested in assisting others to have a child or children they would not otherwise have. The semen provider is being not only acknowledged, but valued for the largely altruistic contribution he makes. He is donating the gift of life.

Many of the semen providers acknowledge the significance of their contribution and see that this has important psychosocial implications for them, the resultant offspring and their parents. Ways of responding to this, especially in terms of the exchange of information, are presenting new and demanding challenges for those most intimately involved as well as for health professionals. There are also important implications for the families and extended networks and for the society of which they are a part. For the latter, the task is to formulate policies which meet the needs and respect the rights of all the parties involved.

REFERENCES

American Fertility Society (1993) 'Guidelines for gamete donation'. *Fertility and Sterility* Supplement 1, 59.
American Fertility Society (Ethics Committee) (1986) 'Ethical considerations of the new reproductive technologies.' *Fertility and Sterility* Supplement 1, 46(3): 36S–38S.
Annas, G. (1980) 'Fathers anonymous: beyond the best interests of the sperm donor'. *Family Law Quarterly* 14: 1–13.
Asche, A. (1985) *Creating children: report of the Family Law Council of Australia.* Canberra: Australian Government Publishing Service.
Austria (1992) *Federal law on medically assisted procreation.* Austria: National Council.
Back, K. W. and Snowden, R. (1988) 'The anonymity of the gamete donor'. *Journal of Psychosomatic Obstetrics and Gynaecology* 9: 191–8.
Baran, A. and Pannor, R. (1989) *Lethal secrets.* New York: Warner Books.
Barratt, C. L. R. (1993) 'Donor recruitment, selection and screening'. In C. L. R. Barratt and I. D. Cooke, eds., *Donor Insemination.* Cambridge: Cambridge University Press, pp. 3–11.
Barratt, C. L. R., Monteiro, E. F., Chauhan, M., and Cooke, S. (1989) 'Screening donors for sexually transmitted disease in donor insemination clinics in the UK. A survey'. *British Journal of Obstetrics and Gynaecology* 96: 461–6.
Beck, W. W. (1984) 'Two hundred years of artificial insemination.' *Fertility and Sterility* 41(2): 193–5.
Bell, C. and Newby, H. (1976) 'Husbands and wives: the dynamics of the deferential dialectic'. In D. L. Barker and S. Allen, eds., *Dependence and Exploitation in Work and Marriage.* New York: Longman, chapter 8.
Blank, R. H. (1990) *Regulating reproduction.* NY: Columbia University Press.
Blood, J. (1992) 'Sperm donors – survey of attitudes to information sharing and maintenance of central register'. Presentation at the XIth Annual Scientific Meeting of the Fertility Society of Australia, Adelaide, 2–5 December.
Bordson, B. L. and Leonardo, V. S. (1991) 'The appropriate upper age limit for semen donors: a review of the genetic effects of paternal age'. *Fertility and Sterility* 56(3): 397–401.
Brandon, J. and Warner, J. (1977) 'AID and adoption: some comparisons'. *British Journal of Social Work* 7(3): 335–41.
Braude, P., Johnson, M. H. and Aitken, R. J. (1990) 'Human fertilisation and embryology bill goes to report stage'. *British Medical Journal* 300: 1,410–12.
British Andrology Society (1993) 'British Andrology Society guidelines for the screening of semen donors for donor insemination'. *Human Reproduction* 8(9): 1,521–3.
British Medical Association (1973) 'Report of Panel on Human Artificial Insemination'. *British Medical Journal* Supplement 3, 2(3).
Chapman, S. P. and Crittenden, J. A. (1992) 'Optimising a donor insemination program: the donor perspective'. Presentation at the XIth Annual Scientific Meeting of the Fertility Society of Australia, Adelaide, 2–5 December.

Chauhan, M., Barratt, C. L. R., Cooke, S. and Cooke, I. D. (1988) 'A protocol for recruitment and screening of semen donors for an artificial insemination by donor programme'. *Human Reproduction* 3(7): 873–6.

Clayton, C. E. and Kovacs, G. T. (1980) 'AID – a pretreatment social assessment'. *Australia and New Zealand Journal of Obstetrics and Gynaecology* 20: 208–10.

Condon, M. and Harrison, K. (1992) 'Sperm donors: attitudes to openness of information to recipient couples'. Presentation at the XIth Annual Scientific Meeting of the Fertility Society of Australia, Adelaide, 2–5 December.

Cook, R. and Golombok, S. (1995) 'A survey of semen donation: phase II – the view of the donors'. *Human Reproduction* 10(4): 951–9.

Curie-Cohen, M., Luttrell, L. and Shapiro, S. (1979) 'Current practice of artificial insemination by donor in the United States'. *New England Journal of Medicine* 300(11): 585–90.

Curson, R. and Daniels, K. (under review) Recruiting semen donors without financial incentives.

Daniels, K. R. (1987) 'Semen donors in New Zealand: their characteristics and attitudes'. *Clinical Reproduction and Fertility* 5(4): 177–90.

(1989) 'Semen donors: their motivations and attitudes to their offspring'. *Journal of Reproductive and Infant Psychology* 7(2): 121–7.

(1993) 'Infertility counselling: the need for a psychosocial perspective'. *British Journal of Social Work* 23(5): 501–15.

(1994) 'The Swedish Insemination Act and its impact'. *Australian and New Zealand Journal of Obstetrics and Gynaecology* 34(4): 437–9.

(1995) 'Information sharing in DI – a conflict of needs and rights'. *Cambridge Quarterly of Healthcare Ethics* 4: 217–24.

Daniels, K. R., Curson, R. and Lewis, G. L. (1996) 'Semen donor recruitment: a study of donors in two clinics'. *Human Reproduction* 11(4): 746–51.

Daniels, K. R., Ericsson, H. L. and Burn, I. P. (1996) 'Families and donor insemination: the views of semen donors'. *The Scandinavian Journal of Social Welfare* 5: 229–37.

(in progress) Motivations of semen donors in a Swedish clinic.

Daniels, K. R. and Lalos, O. (1995) 'The Swedish Insemination Act and the availability of donors'. *Human Reproduction* 10(7): 1,871–4.

Daniels, K. R. and Lewis, G. L. (1996a) 'Donor insemination: the gifting and selling of semen'. *Social Science and Medicine* 42(11): 1,521–36.

(1996b) 'Openness of information in the use of donor gametes: developments in New Zealand'. *Journal of Reproductive and Infant Psychology* 14: 57–68.

Daniels, K. R., Lewis, G. M. and Curson, R. (1997) 'Information sharing in semen donation: the views of donors'. *Social Science and Medicine* 44(5): 673–80.

Daniels, K. R. and Taylor, K. (1993) 'Secrecy and openness in donor insemination'. *Politics & the Life Sciences* 12(2): 155–70.

David, A. and Avidan, D. (1976) 'Artificial insemination by donor: clinical and psychological aspects'. *Fertility and Sterility* 27: 528.

Demack, A. G. (1984) *Report of the Special Committee appointed by the Queensland Government to enquire into the laws relating to artificial insemination, in vitro fertilization and other related matters.* State of Queensland, Australia.

Dewar, J. (1989) 'Fathers in law? The case of AID'. In R. Lee and D. Morgan, eds., *Birthrights: law and ethics at the beginnings of life.* London, Routledge.

Dixon, R. E. and Buttram, V. C. (1976) 'Artificial insemination using donor semen: a review of 171 cases'. *Fertility and Sterility* 27(2): 130–4.

Editorial (1975) 'Artificial insemination (donor)'. *British Medical Journal* 4(5,987): 2–3.

Editorial (1979) 'Artificial insemination for all?' *British Medical Journal* 2: 458.

Fidell, L. S. and Marik, J. (1989) 'Paternity by proxy: artificial insemination with donor sperm'. In J. Offerman-Zuckerberg, ed., New York: Plenum, pp. 93–110.

Finegold, W. J. (1964) *Artificial insemination.* Springfield, Illinois: Charles C. Thomas.

Fisher, R. and Peek, J. (1994) 'Giving up anonymity – socialising gamete donation'. Conference of the European Society for Human Reproduction and Embryology, Brussels.

Fox, R. C. and Swazey, J. P. (1978) *The courage to fail. A social view of organ transplants and dialysis.* Chicago: Chicago University Press.

(1992) *Spare parts: organ replacement in American society.* NY: Oxford University Press.

Glezerman, M. (1981) 'Two hundred and seventy cases of artificial donor insemination: management and results'. *Fertility and Sterility* 35: 180–7.

Glover, J. (Chair) (1989) *Fertility and the family. The Glover Report on reproductive technologies to the European Commission.* London: The Fourth Estate.

Government of Canada (1996) An Act respecting human reproduction and commercial transactions relating to human reproduction. Bill C-47. Ottawa, Canadian Communications Group.

Greenblatt, R. M., Handsfield, H. H., Sayers, M. H. and Holmes, K. K. (1986) 'Screening therapeutic insemination donors for sexually transmitted diseases: overview and recommendations'. *Fertility and Sterility* 46(3): 351–64

Gregoire, A. T. and Mayer, R. C. (1965) 'The impregnators'. *Fertility and Sterility* 16(1): 130–4.

Handelsman, D. J., Dunn, S. M., Conway, A. J., Boylan, L. M. and Jansen, R. P. (1985) 'Psychological and attitudinal profiles in donors for artificial insemination'. *Fertility and Sterility* 43(1): 95–101.

HFEA (1996) Fifth annual report. London: HFEA.

(1993) *Code of Practice.* London: HFEA.

Huerre, P. (1980) 'Psychological aspects of semen donation'. In G. David and W. S. Price, eds., *Human artificial insemination and semen preservation.* New York: Plenum, pp. 461–5.

Hummel, W. P. and Talbert, L. M. (1989) 'Current management of a donor insemination program'. *Fertility and Sterility* 51(6): 919–29.

Johnston, I. (1980) 'The donor'. In C. Wood, J. Leeton and G. Kovacs, eds., *Artificial Insemination by Donor.* Melbourne: Brown Prior Andersen.

Joyce, D. N. (1984) 'The implications of greater openness concerning AID'. In British Agencies for Adoption and Fostering, ed., *AID and After: Papers from BAAF, BASW, and A Scottish Working party.* London, British Agencies for Adoption and Fostering.

Kovacs, G. T., Clayton, C. E. and McGowan, P. (1983) 'The attitudes of semen donors'. *Clinical Reproduction and Fertility* 2(1): 397–9.

Leeton, J. and Backwell, J. (1982) 'A preliminary psychosocial follow-up of parents and their children conceived by artificial insemination by donor (AID)'. *Clinical Reproduction and Fertility* 1: 307–10.

Lui, S. C., Weaver, S. M., Robinson, J., Debono, J., Nieland, M. Killick, S. R. and Hay, D. M. (1995) 'A survey of semen donor attitudes'. *Human Reproduction* 10(1): 234–8.

McGowan, M. P., Baker, H. W., Kovacs, G. T. and Rennie, G. (1983) 'Selection of high fertility donors for artificial insemination programmes'. *Clinical Reproduction and Fertility* 2(4): 269–74.

Mahlstedt, P. P. and Greenfeld, D. A. (1989) 'Assisted reproductive technology with donor gametes: the need for patient preparation'. *Fertility and Sterility* 52(6): 908–14.

Mahlstedt, P. P. and Probasco K. A. (1991) 'Sperm donors: their attitudes toward providing medical and psychosocial information for recipient couples and donor offspring'. *Fertility and Sterility* 56(4): 747–53.

Mauss, M. (1954) *The gift: forms and functions of exchange in archaic societies.* Glencoe, IL: Free Press.

Ministerial Committee on Assisted Human Reproduction (New Zealand) (1994) *Assisted Human Reproduction: Navigating Our Future.* New Zealand Government Print.

Monteiro, E., Spencer, R. C., Barratt, C. L. R., Cooke, S. and Cooke, I. D. (1987) 'Sexually transmitted disease in potential semen donors'. *British Medical Journal* 295 (15 August): 418.

Murray, T. H. (1987) 'Gifts of the body and the needs of strangers'. *Hastings Center Report* 17(2): 30–8.

New York Times (1990) 'Mother accuses sperm bank of a mix-up'. 9 March.
    (1992) 'Four charged in illegal sperm bank'. 27 April.

Nicholas, M. K. and Tyler, J. P. P. (1983) 'Characteristics, attitudes and personalities of AI donors'. *Clinical Reproduction and Fertility* 2(1): 389–96.

Nijs, P. and Rouffa, L. (1975) 'A.I.D. couples: psychological and psychopathological evaluation'. *Andrologia* 7(3): 187–94.

Novaes, S. (1989) 'Giving, receiving, repaying: gamete donors and donor policies in reproductive medicine'. *International Journal of Technology Assessment in Health Care* 5: 639–57.

Paul, J. and Durna, E. (1987) 'Attitudes of sperm donors'. Presentation at the Fertility Society of Australia's Annual Conference, 12 November.

Pedersen, B., Nielsen, F. A., Lauritsen, J. G. (1994) 'Psychosocial aspects of donor insemination. Sperm donors – their motivations and attitudes to artificial insemination'. *Acta Obstetrica et Gynecologica Scandinavica* 73: 701–5

People (1992) 'Betrayal of trust. A fertility doctor is accused of secretly fathering as many as 75 children'. 3 September.

Purdie, A., Peek, J. C., Adair, V., Graham F. and Fisher R. (1994) 'Attitudes of parents of young children to sperm donation – implications for donor recruitment'. *Human Reproduction* 9(7): 1,355–8.

Purdie, A., Peek, J. C. Irwin, R., Graham F. M. and Fisher, P. R. (1992) 'Identifiable semen donors – attitudes of donors and recipient couples'. *New Zealand Medical Journal* 105(927): 27–8.

Rosenkvist, H. (1981) 'Donor insemination'. *Danish Medical Bulletin* 28(4, 1): 133–48.

Rowland, R. (1983) 'Attitudes and opinions of donors on an artificial insemination by donor (AID) programme'. *Clinical Reproduction and Fertility* 2(4): 249–59.

(1985) 'The social and psychological consequences of secrecy in artificial insemination by donor (AID) programmes'. *Social Science and Medicine* 21: 391–6.

Royal Commission on New Reproductive Technologies (Canada) (1993) *Proceed with care, Volume 1*. Minister of Government Services, Ottawa.

Rubin, B. (1965) 'Psychological aspects of human artificial insemination'. *Archives of General Psychiatry* 13: 121–32.

Sauer, M. V., Gorrill, M. J., Zeffer, K. B. and Bustillo, M. (1989) 'Attitudinal survey of sperm donors to an artificial insemination clinic'. *Journal of Reproductive Medicine* 34(5): 362–4.

Schover, L. R., Rothman, S. A. and Collins, R. L. (1992) 'The personality and motivation of semen donors: a comparison with oocyte donors'. *Human Reproduction* 7(4): 575–9.

Schoysman, R. (1975) 'Problems of selecting donors for artificial insemination'. *Journal of Medical Ethics* 1(1): 34–5.

Schroeder-Jenkins, M. and Rothmann, S. A. (1989) 'Causes of donor rejection in a sperm banking program'. *Fertility and Sterility* 51(5): 903–6.

Selva, J., Leonard, C., Albert, M., Auger, J. and David, G. (1986) 'Genetic screening for artificial insemination by donor (AID)'. *Clinical Genetics* 29: 389–96.

Snowden, R., Mitchell, G. D. and Snowden, E. (1983) *Artificial reproduction: a social investigation*. London: Allen and Unwin.

Stacey, M. (1992) 'Social dimensions of assisted reproduction'. In M. Stacey, ed., *Changing human reproduction. Social science perspectives*. London: Sage Publications, pp. 9–47.

Strathern, M. (1992) 'The meaning of assisted kinship'. In M. Stacey, ed., *Changing Human reproduction. Social science perspectives*. London: Sage Publications, pp. 148–69.

Strickler, R. C., Keller, D. W. and Warren, J. C. (1975) 'Artificial insemination with fresh donor semen'. *New England Journal of Medicine* 293(17): 848–53.

Sweden (1984) *Swedish Law on Artificial Insemination, 1140/1984*. Swedish Parliament.

Titmuss, R. M. (1970) *The gift relationship: from human blood to social policy.* Harmondsworth: Pelican.

Victorian State Parliament (Australia) (1995) *Infertility Treatment Bill 1995*. Melbourne: L. V. North, Government Printer.

Warnock, M. (1984) *Report of the Committee of Inquiry into Human Fertilisation and Embryology*. Department of Health and Social Security. London: HMSO.

Worsnop, D., Mack, H., Robbie, A., Song, L. Y. and McGuire, P. (1982) 'Human artificial insemination: donors in Melbourne. From our medical schools'. *Australian Family Physician* 11(3): 218–24.

6 The medical management of donor insemination

Simone Bateman Novaes

Introduction

Medical assistance with conception cannot be explained away as merely another technical achievement due to progress in biology and medicine. An unorthodox approach to the problem of infertility, it has radically altered the usual framework of bodily practices and social relationships which organise and give meaning to reproduction in our society. Until two centuries ago, a birth had always been the result of sexual intercourse between two persons of the opposite sex, whose relationship was already (or, as a consequence of this event, would come to be) defined in familial terms. The use of assisted conception transfers the act of fertilisation to a medical setting, where relationships are primarily defined in therapeutic terms, where predominant values concern the quality, security and efficiency of a technical act, and where the physician is held responsible for the appropriate management of medical procedures. Decisions are now being made about childbearing in a context which dissociates issues relating to fertility and the family from sexual intercourse.

The more recent extracorporeal technique known as *in vitro* fertilisation has made it seem obvious that assistance with conception necessarily involves medical intervention: without physicians to monitor hormonal stimulation, perform laparoscopy or ultrasound probes for oocyte retrieval, and place *in vitro* fertilised embryos within the uterus, such a technique would in fact not be possible. However, the much older and simpler technique, known as artificial insemination does not require such medical intervention: it is fairly simple to find the adequate instrumental means for transferring semen to the vagina.[1] This raises the question as to why physicians have none the less been consistently involved in this practice.

Assisted conception is far from being standard medical treatment for infertility. On the contrary, these techniques tend presently to be used when all attempts to address the cause of an individual's infertility problem by drugs or surgical procedures have failed. Their rationale is to circumvent the obstacles to conception through sexual intercourse, by using alternative instrumental means to produce a pregnancy. Insofar as many forms of medical treatment address symptoms rather than causes, medical assistance with fertilisation can eventually be said to treat infertility in that it does try to deal with what may be seen as infertility's major symptom: childlessness. None the less, the therapeutic attributes of these procedures seem to have more to do with the stigma of childlessness than with the physical ailments which are at its source. Assisted conception thus presents itself essentially as a medically managed solution to a painful personal and social problem.

What reasoning led physicians to assume that they were providing treatment for infertility, when the technical act they were proposing may be understood as an alternative mode of conception to heterosexual intercourse? When physicians are confronted with an infertility problem, they usually have to deal with two constraints: one was, and still is, the limits of scientific knowledge and effective medical solutions to the problem of infertility; the other was, but appears less so today, a moral and social question regarding the propriety of his/her intervention in sexual and reproductive matters. These domains are today defined as being within the limits of a physician's professional competence, but it must be remembered that, at the end of the eighteenth century, the presence of a (male) physician at childbirth was still a rare event, exceptionally justified by their monopoly of a new instrument, the forceps, designed to facilitate difficult births. Thus the possibility of providing some form of *technical* assistance with reproductive processes, even if of an experimental nature, may have been perceived outright by physicians as sufficient to justify interfering in their patients' reproductive concerns.

The fact that assisted conception, despite its peculiar characteristics, is now generally accepted as a form of *medical treatment* for infertility, has given physicians crucial leverage in decision-making with respect to many, if not most, aspects of these practices. They have managed to impose their perception of the way infertility should be handled and have often defined the situations in which such treatment may be legitimately provided. As gatekeepers, they have frequently brought to closure social and moral issues of reproductive choice which would normally require collective debate. Understanding medical involvement in assisted conception, beyond those aspects related to technical competence, thus becomes a key element in grasping the profound changes in our procreative attitudes and behaviour brought about by these techniques.

Insemination, with or without donor semen, is one of the oldest and simplest forms of medically assisted conception. From the first experimental attempts with animals by Lazzaro Spallanzani in the eighteenth century to the more recent widespread development of DI organised around semen banks, its long history illustrates how physicians have come to be considered professionally competent in matters pertaining to conception. This chapter, which focuses mainly on the medical management of DI, will try to show how instrumental insemination (with or without donor semen) came to be constructed as treatment for male infertility; how new therapeutic relationships and institutional structures have resulted from the medical provision of such treatment; how the constructs which shape medical practice respond to concerns with the social and moral legitimacy of instrumental insemination; and how the problems and conflicts encountered in daily practice have raised unexpected questions concerning medical responsibility and patient autonomy in decisions concerning procreative matters. Special attention will be given to semen banking: by making DI a more socially visible practice and bringing the major issues related to the moral and social legitimacy of such a practice out into the open, it has set the scene for the development of fertilisation techniques, with increased acceptance (if not demand) of medical intervention in reproductive matters.

The construction of donor insemination as medical treatment

Attempts to develop adequate treatment for male infertility have encountered numerous obstacles over the years. Many factors require consideration: the production and the maturing of sperm in the male genital apparatus involve complex hormonal mechanisms; fertilisation in the female body requires that there be no anatomical, neurological or psychological obstacles to ejaculation; male fertility must also be evaluated relative to that of the female partner (men with a low sperm count may in fact engender offspring with no problems, if their partner is especially fertile). Although progress has been made in identifying some of the causes of male infertility, the origins of many conditions still elude fertility specialists. Diagnostic techniques have improved, but efficient therapeutic procedures concern only very few conditions (Finegold 1976; Kunstmann 1979; Novaes 1994a).

However, many physicians who have long been involved in the treatment of infertility have expressed the feeling that, until recent times, the most formidable and long-lasting of these obstacles has probably been cultural in nature: men find it difficult to accept (when they do not deny) that the cause of an infertility problem might be related to a male physiological factor.[2] Whereas women have almost always been ready to submit to drastic diagnostic work-ups and treatment in the hopes of being able to bear a child, the suggestion that their husband or partner might need to be brought in for medical examination and treatment was often met by the partner's outright refusal. Progress in the treatment of male infertility has therefore also had to take into account male susceptibility concerning any problem too closely related to sexual potency and identity.

The idea that assisted conception reflects a contemporary revolution in infertility treatment is misleading in that it tends to neglect some historical facts: it must be remembered that experimentation with instrumental fertilisation dates back to the end of the eighteenth century. At the time, biological science was beginning to develop knowledge through experiments which attempted to replicate naturally-occurring phenomena under laboratory circumstances: this may explain the idea of approaching the problem of infertility by an instrumental imitation of copulation (da Silva 1991). With respect to reproduction, there was heated debate as to whether an individual entity originated from the egg or from the 'little animals' (sperm) in semen, and whether it existed as a totally preformed entity since the beginning of times or whether it developed gradually from a few initial cells. The abbot and scientist Lazzaro Spallanzani (1729–1799) was deeply involved in this debate and was paradoxically trying to devise experiments which might contribute conclusive evidence in support of the theory that the future individual existed totally preformed in the female egg. After experimenting with different elements of external fertilisation in frogs and successfully obtaining the birth of live animals through artificial insemination of a female dog in heat, he was able to conclude that contact between semen and the female egg(s) was necessary for fertilisation to take place; only the role of the 'little animals' in semen remained unclear (Mayr 1982; Giordan 1987; da Silva 1991).

If contact between semen and eggs was necessary for fertilisation to take place, was it also sufficient? According to one of Spallanzani's contemporaries, the Swiss abbot Jean Senebier, Spallanzani's experiment with the dog resulted in the birth of several animals 'whose conception could not be imputed to the cooperation of a male' (Senebier, quoted in da Silva 1991). It is probably the absence of a physically present male involved in a sexual act with the female, that leads him to this unusual conclusion, which also does not take into account the act Spallanzani himself performed for fertilisation to occur. However, this statement might also be explained by the idea that orgasm and thus coition was long thought to be indispensable to conception (Laqueur 1990). Whereas what was happening on the cellular level still remained obscure to eighteenth-century scientists, it is the fact that sexual intercourse was not a necessary condition to fertilisation that most struck their scientific imagination. Spallanzani's experiments thus seem primarily to have established that a pregnancy could be generated by 'imitating nature',[3] that is, by using alternative means to sexual intercourse to transfer semen from a man's to a woman's body.

The results of these experiments appear to have inspired physicians, who began using instrumental insemination at about this time: the first recorded cases, by John Hunter in England and by M. A. Thouret in France, date back to the turn of the nineteenth century. The technique seems to have been an attempt to elude anatomical obstructions to fertilisation through sexual intercourse,[4] but also to circumvent sexual difficulties resulting in childlessness, or simply to avoid the 'inconveniences' of intercourse[5] (Home 1799; Thouret 1803; Kunstmann 1979). Practised discreetly during the first half of the nineteenth century, the procedure later became extremely popular and extraordinary claims were made about its results; these, in fact, seem hardly possible, as inseminations were often practiced during menstruation, thought at the time to be the most fertile moment of a woman's reproductive cycle (Finegold 1976; Kunstmann 1979; Snowden and Mitchell 1981; David 1986, 1991).

The practice of instrumental insemination developed and began to be advocated as a therapeutic procedure, but it ultimately met with reactions of strong disapproval. Representatives of the medical hierarchy expressed doubts and criticism regarding what they considered indiscriminate use of the technique. Moreover, in the light of religiously inspired sexual codes, the physician's instrumental substitution of sexual intercourse was far from being seen as medically justified or as morally excusable; the fact that masturbation was required to provide semen made the practice all the more suspect. In France, the first public condemnation of instrumental insemination pronounced at a trial in Bordeaux brings moral charges to bear on the practice: it 'was offensive to natural law, could constitute a real social peril, and it was of import to the dignity of marriage that such procedures not be transferred from the domain of Science to that of Practice' (Tribunal de Bordeaux, 1880, Affaire Lejâtre, cited by David, 1986: 204). As early as 1897, the Vatican also condemned instrumental insemination as a violation of natural law, and has since systematically reiterated this position (most recently, in an instruction from the Vatican, *Donum vitae*, 1987, and in the encyclical *Evangelium vitae*, 1995).

None the less, knowledge about different aspects of fertility and conception, including the respective roles of egg and sperm in fertilisation, was pursued and increased considerably during the second half of the nineteenth century. New findings about fertilisation at the cellular level allowed for the idea that the male factor in infertility might also be due to problems with the quality of the semen itself. Some physicians began to experiment with methods for improving the husband's semen (Kunstmann 1979), and in the United States, in 1884 (as revealed in an article published in 1909) a physician named Pancoast attempted replacing the husband's apparently unproductive semen by that of another, supposedly more fertile, man (Gregoire and Mayer 1965). DI proved to be a more effective remedy than insemination with the husband's own semen. However, this way of proceeding suggested adultery, with all the social, psychological and moral objections that such conduct raised, as well as the legal paternity problems that might ensue; it could thus only foment the hostile climate which already surrounded instrumental insemination.

The controversial nature of this unorthodox medical procedure led to the reinforcement of a perceived need for discretion, particularly in those circumstances in which physicians resorted to an anonymous semen provider.[6] Even in the United States, where the Catholic Church's view on natural law had far less influence on moral questions than on parts of the European continent, Dr J. Marion Sims, having himself reported fifty-five instrumental inseminations performed on six women, ultimately abandoned the procedure for moral reasons (Finegold 1976: 6); as for Pancoast's successful experiment with donor semen, it was kept a secret for twenty-five years. If DI was sometimes discussed in the English language medical literature, there was no public mention of it in France until 1949, at which time, the French Academy for Moral and Political Sciences formally condemned the practice. This view was reiterated at a meeting of the Federation of French-speaking Societies of Gynaecology and Obstetrics, organized in 1957 on the theme of the 'Medical and social study of artificial insemination'. The historical origins of assisted conception are clearly tainted by doubts about the morality of the acts involved and their legitimacy as medical treatment (Finegold 1976; Kunstmann 1979; David 1986, 1991).

New therapeutic relationships, new institutional structures

As long as instrumental insemination remained an exceptional response to the problem of male infertility, secrecy could be considered the simplest and most effective way of handling the social and moral objections raised against this procedure. Women whose husbands could not be treated successfully, were inseminated during a private consultation with the semen from a fertile man, usually in exchange for small monetary compensation. In the case of DI, evidence in support of paternity suits could be avoided by concealing the identity of the semen provider and by not keeping files on the procedure and its results.[7] (See chapter by Daniels in this volume.) These measures guaranteed discretion and allowed the couple and their children to appear to others as a 'normally' constituted family (Snowden and Mitchell 1981). However, they did not ensure that (as might be expected of a medical procedure) the medical acts performed and their results would be subject to rigorous evaluation and control.

The conditions under which the three principal participants of DI (the woman to be inseminated, the man providing the semen, and the physician) were being brought together, emphasised the moral premises of this arrangement: even if the offer of treatment might ultimately be justifiable in terms of its positive results, it was nevertheless not perceived as morally appropriate or legally expedient for the infertile couple to be acquainted with the semen provider. The physician therefore, beyond his/her technical role as inseminator, had to intervene as a mediator: someone who makes it possible for semen transfer to take place, without requiring the two parties to meet. Secrecy surrounding the procedure and the anonymity of the semen provider became the primary organising principles of the practice, and in a certain sense served as the most obvious justification for the physician's presence in this situation[8] (Novaes 1994a).

The advent of semen banking in the second half of the twentieth century considerably changes certain aspects of this initial scenario. The main participants are no longer brought together at the same place and at approximately the same time: the fact that semen can be frozen makes it possible to deal with semen providers quite independently of any particular request for DI. This allows for an expansion in time and space of the circuit established between the different protagonists, and introduces a novel complexity into the circuit, particularly at the new locus, the semen bank, where mediation between semen providers and recipients is taking place.

But what in fact is a semen bank? Understood in its simplest form as a technical object, it is a metallic container in which straws, containing semen prepared with a cryoprotective medium, are kept frozen in liquid nitrogen (at about $-191°C$). Physicians may have such a 'bank' in their private offices where they perform inseminations, without having themselves been responsible for the preparation of the straws it contains. From a sociological perspective, it is therefore preferable to restrict the use of the term *semen bank* to laboratory facilities ensuring the preparation, stocking and distribution of frozen semen. This helps bring to the fore the now more complex network of participants involved in DI, making it possible to examine the impact on relationships among participants of a change in technical procedure.[9]

In a semen bank, the physician is in fact no longer the sole protagonist in a mediating position: semen banking multiplies the number of interrelated actors organising the transfer of semen. At the very least, the freezing and storing of semen require the presence of qualified laboratory technicians, and managing daily business with clients implies that one or more physicians (depending on the size of the facilities) receive and screen semen providers and respond to requests for frozen semen. Secretarial help is indispensable, not only for contact with clients, but also for help in maintaining files of medical and personal information, some of which is codified to remain anonymous. Semen banks may also sometimes collaborate directly with physicians practising inseminations, with geneticists special-ised in screening semen providers (and even eventually recipients), or with psychologists capable of providing help with the emotional problems of infertility. The laboratory facility may or may not be a part of a larger clin-ical service specialising in infertility.

In this more elaborate organisation of the practice of DI, no individual physician is any longer in a position *immediately and directly* to negotiate and arrange the anonymous transfer of semen from one party to the other. Each physician is now subjected to fewer situational constraints in dealing with the specific problems of each party and may thus bring to bear, in selecting semen providers or in choosing a semen sample for a particular recipient, medical criteria which the morally ambiguous climate and the time pressure of the preceding circumstances made difficult to apply. Practical conditions now favour the evaluation and quality control of pro-cedures, which begin to emerge as a deontologically necessary concern.

Semen banks, thus defined as a laboratory facility, did not appear in any systematic manner until the 1970s. The cryopreservation of semen and semen banking were technically possible as early as 1949; however, the use of cryopreserved semen was for a long time restricted essentially to the insemination of bovines. Ten years later, banks for human semen did crop up, essentially in Japan and the United States, but for the most part as com-mercial ventures providing 'fertility insurance' for men who were to undergo vasectomy: were these men, at a later date and under different cir-cumstances, to wish once again to have children, this would hypothetically be possible through insemination with their cryopreserved semen. One of the pioneers in the area of cryobiology, Jerome K. Sherman, made many efforts to promote semen banking, which he also hoped would provide the necessary conditions for development of research in reproductive biology (Sherman 1964, 1973).[10] However, the banking of human semen did not fare well, as long as its major purposes revolved around the commercial exploitation of self-imposed infertility: demand for this type of service was insufficient and the reliability of such 'insurance' was frequently questioned (Sherman 1964, 1973; Frankel 1973; David 1991).

Semen banking did none the less finally take root, but in another country: France. These cryopreservation facilities were set up for the most part on a non-commercial basis and with a different objective: re-organis-ing the practice of DI. The configuration of daily practice did not exclude opportunities for research in reproductive biology and epidemiology, but the main concern of the founders of these banks was to offer their patients a better quality medical service than that which could be obtained in the quasi-clandestine conditions of existing practices of DI.

At the origin of French semen banks were two physicians, Georges David, a specialist in the biology of sperm, and Albert Netter, a gynaecologist. Both were regularly confronted with the problem of male infertility and decided at about the same time to propose DI to their patients in what they conceived of as an institutionally more adequate framework. Contrary to what might be expected, neither of these physicians had any previous experience with cryobiology. However, it is precisely because, as physicians, they were confronted with the emotional distress of patients for whom they could offer no effective form of treatment, that the idea of using semen banks to organise a commendable practice of DI came up as a possible alternative.

Two characteristics are peculiar to the French conception of semen banking: the first is its quasi-monopolistic position in recruiting and selecting semen providers and in distributing cryopreserved donor semen for insemination. To practitioners in most other countries, the use of cryopreserved semen for DI remained for a long time only an occasional alternative to the preferred option of semen provided fresh at the time of insemination. With fresh semen, there is in fact a higher probability of obtaining a pregnancy in any given cycle than with frozen. The appearance of the AIDS virus, however, with a few cases of contamination by insemination, greatly influenced a change of attitudes: frozen semen can be quarantined until the provider has been retested, three to six months later, and found negative for the AIDS virus (US Congress, Office of Technology Assessment 1988). In France, the use of cryopreserved semen immediately appeared as a preferable option, particularly to Professor Georges David, the founder of what later became a nation-wide network of semen banks, CECOS (Centre d'Etude et de Conservation des Oeufs et du Sperme humains). This was precisely because it was perceived outright as allowing for a more thorough control of the health of semen providers, as well as providing the conditions necessary for an improvement in the standards of practice of artificial insemination.

In fact, the second characteristic peculiar to the French system is the control of medical indications for insemination. In many countries, semen banks simply provide an alternative source of donor semen, distributed according to specifications determined by the physicians attending to a request for DI. In France, the actual performance of inseminations was and still is most often left to physicians in the private sector; bank physicians more rarely perform inseminations, and only if the bank is associated or contiguous to clinical services. However, physicians in the private sector must always refer their patients to bank physicians for the dispensing of frozen semen. The bank physicians may occasionally disagree with the referring physician and recommend a supplementary work-up or just more patience before involving a couple in DI or any other form of assisted conception. Bank physicians usually also require that the data concerning the insemination procedure be relayed back to them, both for control of results and for epidemiological research purposes. All in all, they are the ones who ultimately decide whether or not cryopreserved semen should be dispensed to a particular couple: a situation which may sometimes create tension and conflict, not only with the couples but with the referring physician.

DI thus set up as a practice organised around semen banking quickly began to shed its quasi-clandestine and ambiguous therapeutic status, particularly in France. It became a more socially visible and apparently more respectable procedure, now openly mediated by physicians in an institutionally stable management position. As in preceding circumstances, physicians in a mediating position are the only participants in the circuit to have access to information concerning both parties; this, of course, already gives them crucial decision-making power over other participants in the circuit. The advent of semen banking made it possible for physicians to create the necessary technical and social conditions to review and improve their standards of practice and, by this very fact, they have found themselves in a privileged position to impose their professional views and values as a perspective validated by experience in organizing the practice and evaluating its consequences.

Despite these major transformations in the practice of DI, semen banking has not changed at least one fundamental element: the moral rationale underlying the relationships among protagonists in DI. Keeping semen providers and the woman being inseminated from meeting each other remains a constant preoccupation and, as we have seen, semen banking simply makes it technically easier to deal with this major factor of unease for all the participants involved. Most countries have maintained anonymity and secrecy as organising principles (Haimes 1990, 1992; Novaes 1994a), when they have not made them legal requirements.[11] Paradoxically, however, more persons have come to share in the secrets of DI and society is now more openly informed that this practice exists. Sweden's recent laws regulating DI and doing away with non-identifiable semen providers (Ewerlöf 1985; Hamberger 1986; Daniels 1994b), as well as trends in this direction in countries such as Australia and New Zealand (Handelsman et al. 1985; Daniels 1988, 1989, 1994a; Purdie et al. 1992), seem to indicate that prevailing attitudes towards DI, particularly with regards to the moral and social issues it raises, could be changing.

Constructing the legitimacy of medical mediation

The history of assisted conception (until the mid-twentieth century, essentially the history of assisted insemination) points to a major question raised by this approach to infertility: is the instrumental (i.e. non-sexual) transfer of gametes a morally acceptable and socially legitimate procreative practice? This complex question articulates moral issues regarding reproductive choices to public policy issues about regulation, but both have been traditionally obscured by the fact that the social entrenchment of an instrumental approach to conception has been constructed for the most part in medical terms. For many years, these issues were almost never openly addressed, let alone answered: the hostile climate which surrounded instrumental insemination seemed clearly to indicate that the practice should not be pursued. Some physicians none the less did, and ultimately tried to tackle the deontological issues raised by the medicalisation of an instrumental procreative procedure.

From the beginning, the very presence and interference of physicians in this area was questioned: what entitles a physician to intervene in a patient's problems with fertility, which were, until the turn of the nineteenth century, perceived as matters exclusively related to religious questions and to one's private sexual life? Physicians who, despite general hostility, agreed to become involved in their patients' concerns about childbearing, probably did so because new scientific dicoveries may have made them feel (and led them to be perceived as) both technically competent and professionally qualified to be entrusted with a morally delicate problem concerning one's body. By authorizing themselves to provide even an experimental form of treatment in an attempt to find an effective solution to their patients' problems, physicians were in fact beginning, there and then, to construct the legitimacy of both the technical act and their presence in this unorthodox therapeutic scenario. None the less, transforming DI into more than an occasional secretive practice ultimately required that they openly confront the principal moral and legal objections to instrumental insemination, revolving mainly around the fact that semen was being provided under circumstances associated with adulterous conduct.

Two separate problems needed to be addressed: on one hand, the legitimacy of the paternity established by DI in favour of the infertile husband of the inseminated woman; on the other, the legitimacy of the different aspects of the medical practice itself, including the very offer of 'treatment'.

The first question does not really lie within the scope of this chapter, and mainly for this reason, I will not deal with it here. Moreover, the legal provisions relating to paternity are sometimes quite different from one country to another and it would be difficult to generalize from any one particular case. (See the chapter by Blank in this collection.) However, it is important to note that, in some countries (and this has been particularly true in France[12]), physicians themselves have often contributed to the political pressure for legislation clarifying the situation; for in fact, the legality of the kinship relationships established by DI is a fundamental element conferring legitimacy to the practice itself.

None the less, the legitimacy of *medical* interference with problems related to conception, whether or not donor gametes are involved, cannot rest entirely on legal provisions regulating the attribution of parental status. It must somehow be warranted by the inherent characteristics of the situation. Physicians have tended to justify their presence in a reproductive scenario, not by their technical competence to perform a procedure (which in the case of DI cannot be argued), but by defining an area of legitimate professional expertise which accounts for interference with conception, while setting conditions and limits to such interference, based on the principles of good medical practice. In everyday situations, however, as apparently medical criteria are brought into play, the coherence of their deontological position is constantly being undermined by the moral, social and cultural issues at stake in the practice.

These often unprecedented practical situations refer physicians back to what, still today, remains an unanswered question: is instrumental insemination as such an acceptable procreative alternative to sexual intercourse? Medicalisation of the procedure has tended to frame this issue in slightly different terms, suggesting that the answer to the preceding question may be negative: under what conditions and circumstances may assisted conception be legitimately provided? Constructs shaping medical practice are an attempt to offer a pertinent response to this question.

Access to 'treatment'. The increasing visibility of assisted conception has confronted physicians with an unforeseen problem: their prospective clients are no longer only married (or unmarried) couples with infertility problems, but also women with requests unrelated to infertility. In countries where there are more positive cultural attitudes towards childbearing outside of the heterosexual family structure, physicians tend to be more tolerant about requests from single women or from lesbian couples (Englert 1994). However, in many countries, physicians feel that they should not respond to these types of requests and justify their refusal of treatment on the basis that, in these particular situations, there is no *medical* reason for them to intervene (Shenfield 1994). After all, these women are fertile and could have children 'normally' with any fertile male partner. In other words, many physicians feel they cannot legitimately provide instrumental assistance with conception if the sole reason is to short-circuit the circumstances which require sexual intercourse: the woman to be inseminated must have an infertile male partner within a socially recognized reproductive relationship. These physicians have thus tended for the most part to restrict their provision of reproductive services to patients for whom such treatment is 'medically indicated', that is, to cases in which a physiological obstacle or cause prevents conception under the usual circumstances (Novaes 1994a). These restrictive attitudes are often reflected in legislation.[13]

For many physicians, the notion of a medical indication is a reassuring limit to a practice perceived as capable of leading them far beyond the boundaries of medical treatment as such. This is particularly true of physicians involved with DI which, more often than other techniques, is solicited by women desiring to become parents in the absence of a partner of the other sex or even after their partner's death. The sense of security provided by the notion of a medical indication is nevertheless illusory, in that it does not take into consideration the complexity of the practical situations to which this medical construct leads.

The very notion of a medical indication for DI cannot be treated as a technical construct as such: a medical indication appears rather as a practical normative construct in which medical and social justifications are woven together, in this case precisely because only women, whose husbands or male partners are – for whatever reason – infertile, may have access to treatment. And even as a technical construct, the notion of a medical indication is not a clearly defined limit. Indications for DI may range from various types of problems with sperm (insufficient number or motility, pathological forms), to anatomical obstructions or sexual obstacles in either the male or the female partner, to various immunological problems (sperm antibodies, cervical mucus hostility). Moreover, the criteria defining an indication are constantly evolving and must be reviewed in the light of the latest scientific knowledge and technical developments, as these may offer unexpected alternative options for treatment.[14]

As physicians refine medical criteria defining an indication and decide, often alone, what is the best response to a particular problem, they may encounter unprecedented situations in which it may no longer be quite clear whether they should be providing treatment, despite the legitimacy of the social relationship of their patients. For example, can the risk of transmitting to the child a serious hereditary condition (such as Huntington's chorea) or even a sexually transmitted disease (such as AIDS) through the partner's semen be considered a valid indication for DI? Is the notion of infertility treatment still pertinent in these cases, as both partners in these situations are fertile? And should one consider infertile, in the usual sense of the term, a heterosexual couple in which one of the partners is a transsexual? To none of these questions is there a strictly technical answer. Physicians are none the less constantly searching for ways to devise a valid medical framework within which they may comfortably respond to the social and cultural questions raised by their unorthodox therapeutic stance.

Semen provider selection. Concern with standards of practice also ultimately creates new problems for provider selection. In the past, the secretive circumstances of insemination meant that, at most, the semen provider would have received a cursory examination of his general health and maybe of his semen; at the very least, he would have been chosen for his healthy appearance. The possibility of freezing semen now allows physicians more time to examine the medical history and the physical condition of a prospective semen provider, as well as the fertilising quality of his sperm.

There has come to be a relative consensus as to the pertinent medical criteria for the selection of semen providers (at least, a medical and family history of the provider is always taken, and the sperm is examined for its fertilising capacity and cultured to control for the eventual presence of germs). There may however be wide variation in the number of examinations carried out and the extent to which verifications are made. In fact, as knowledge increases, particularly with respect to genetics, and as new diagnostic techniques become available, it becomes crucial to determine not only minimum but also maximum standards for selecting a healthy semen provider. Insufficient screening may be considered irresponsible medical conduct, in that it ignores the possibility of transmission of infectious and inherited disease through sperm; excessive selection standards, on the other hand, raise questions as to whether screening is limited to disease prevention, and if not, what other criteria are being used and with what justifications. This problem is particularly critical in the case of genetic screening, as it raises the question as to whether such practices reflect a conventional prophylactic stance in medicine or whether they may be considered eugenic.[15]

Semen providers are selected, in most countries, strictly on criteria related to their physical health and appearance; usually no other particular requirements are expressed (although they may implicitly affect an individual physician's judgement in evaluating a prospective donor). In the French CECOS banks, the semen provider must also possess certain social characteristics: he is expected to be married (or living in a stable relationship), the father of at least one child, and must have his wife's or partner's consent to donation, and he is asked to donate his sperm (as he will receive no monetary compensation). These requirements, a peculiarity of the French system, are often criticised: there are no medical justifications for them[16] and they discriminate against unmarried men without partners or children who might wish to be donors. The absence of payment has also been controversial for pragmatic reasons, as it does reduce the number of donors. This policy has however been upheld as a means of providing anxious recipients with a non-identifying but reassuring portrait of the man behind the anonymous semen provider. It also compels the prospective donor, and those who are recruiting him, to focus some attention on the possible effects of this decision on his own personal life.[17] Of course, this cannot be expected to be a cost effective procedure, as it makes donor recruitment more difficult and allows for self-exclusion on the basis of non-medical reasons (Novaes 1989, 1994a, 1994b).

On the other hand, requiring anonymity of the semen provider has, until recently, never appeared as a problematic element in the process of selection: it has always been a self-evident principle of DI and, for the most part, semen providers expected (or were thought to expect) this. However, two new factors seem to be pressing for a change in the traditional DI scenario. The first is concern in certain countries about the importance of knowing one's biological origins: this is argued either from a psychological perspective, related to questions about identity, or in view of recent developments in the area of genetics occasionally making such information medically indispensable. The second is the newer practice of egg donation through *in vitro* fertilisation, which requires the donor to undergo far greater constraints and risks: some have considered it unreasonable and ultimately unacceptable to expect a woman to do this for someone she does not know. Both discussions have contributed to an on-going debate about the unquestioned validity of the principle of anonymity.

Sweden is the first country legally to require that the identity of semen providers be on register, for future reference in the case of a request from persons born by DI. In a few countries, such as the United States (Jacobs 1993; Seligman 1995) and New Zealand (Purdie *et al.* 1992), a prospective donor occasionally has the option, in certain infertility services, of agreeing to provide semen under conditions which allow for his future identification by offspring born from use of his semen. Quite obviously, access to the identity of the semen provider supposes that parents of persons born by this procedure will have communicated this fact to them. Present attitudes towards DI remain ambivalent and thus make this far from certain (Ewerlöf 1985; Hamberger 1986; Daniels 1994b; Daniels *et al.* 1995). (See chapter by Daniels in this collection.)

Matching semen providers and recipients. Once the semen providers have been selected and the couples given access to treatment, a crucial phase in the medical management of DI involves matching semen providers with recipients and deciding what criteria should be used. This in many ways is the phase that both defines and characterizes DI: the partners are not to meet and are not expected to become a socially recognized procreative relationship. As a form of mate matching for temporary procreative purposes, making the decision to pair off two persons, usually unknown to each other and expected to remain so, must pursue a logic of its own. This is why another important question is: who is to make that decision?

In many countries, given the anonymous status of the transaction, choosing a semen provider for a particular recipient is, in most situations, the physician's decision. The criteria, of course, may be highly variable from one situation to another. Physicians using fresh semen have most probably always kept their requirements to a minimum, in that they are always necessarily constrained by the question of a man's availability at the appropriate time. The secrecy which, until recent times, almost always protected their practice from indiscrete investigations allows for few indications as to what these criteria might be (Curie-Cohen *et al.* 1979). For semen bank physicians, the semen provider's availability is no longer a problem: they have at their disposal a stock of cryopreserved semen from different men, thus giving them a wider spectrum of choice. However, as DI, constructed as medical treatment, becomes a more socially visible practice, there will be general expectation that criteria for matching providers and recipients be consistent, publicly known and open to discussion. The latter expectations are met, in part, by the leaflets which present the practice to future semen providers and recipients, as well as by the publication of practice standards and results in medical journals.

The criteria most often mentioned by physicians for matching semen providers and recipients are: blood type and diverse morphological criteria related to physical appearance (colour of the skin, hair, and eyes; height and weight). The argument justifying a choice according to these criteria is usually that the semen provider should resemble the infertile male partner or, in a finer version of this argument which takes into account the genetics of reproduction, should have hereditary traits which, mingled with those of the woman to be inseminated, make it plausible that the child born from this match is the male partner's offspring. Quite obviously, although the criteria are physical characteristics, the reasoning on which the matching is based is fundamentally social:[18] specific traits of the semen provider should disappear in the child, so as not to disturb the fragile equilibrium between the two partners in constituting and bringing up their family. Despite the social visibility and apparent legitimacy of DI as a medical practice, secrecy about the social effects and consequences of this procedure remains an essential preoccupation in the matching of traits.

Some physicians, usually a minority and not in all countries, may take into account both provider and recipient preference with respect to the choice of a semen provider. A physician may eventually accept a 'personal donor', that is a relative or a friend of the persons requesting DI and who agrees to donate his semen for their exclusive use. More often though, such arrangements are made without resorting to a physician. Some physicians and semen banks give recipients the option of choosing an 'identifiable donor', that is, a semen provider who accepts the principle of having his identity revealed to adult offspring born from use of his semen (Purdie *et al.* 1992; Jacobs 1993; Seligman 1995). In most cases, however, semen providers are expected (or often still choose) to remain anonymous, but they do sometimes allow (or would at least permit) physicians to reveal a certain number of distinguishing personal traits and preferences, as well as elements regarding their social status, allowing recipients to make a choice on the basis of their own personal and cultural preferences (Handelsman *et al.* 1985; Jacobs 1993; Daniels 1988, 1989). In all of these circumstances, the reasoning underlying matching is more overtly social: it promotes as a value the recipient's freedom to make a personal reproductive choice, limited eventually only by the precautions expected of any good medical practitioner. In principle, the physician is clearly opting not to interfere with decisions related to personal reproductive preferences. (See chapter by Daniels in this volume.)

Such arrangements question the therapeutic stance on which DI has so far been constructed and which in fact has tended to establish physicians in a position as gatekeepers on sensitive social issues regarding the family and the welfare of the child. In fact, by opening the concept of assisted conception to provider and recipient preference, physicians seem to be abandoning the notion of DI as treatment, and possibly even relinquishing a professional duty and prerogative, justified by medical training and technical competence, to make major treatment decisions, the consequences for which they must assume professional responsibility. Some physicians are critical of what appears as a more permissive practice, incompatible with the deontological requirements of the profession and perilous in its consequences for the welfare of the child (Jalbert *et al.* 1989; Shenfield 1994).

Can assisted conception, open to provider and recipient preference, still be considered a *medical* procedure and if so, in what respect? If it is not, why have some physicians nevertheless set up their practice in this way? There are many ways of addressing this issue, and it would be far too easy to find deontologically at fault all of those physicians allowing for donor or recipient preference. If one cannot exclude that this may eventually be the case for some of them, it too conveniently puts aside what may in fact be one of the major unresolved issues underlying the moral and social rationale of DI.

Professional responsibility and reproductive decisions

As DI is now widely perceived as infertility treatment, the conditions and limits of legitimate medical interference in reproductive decisions are rarely considered a public issue, to be examined as such (Novaes 1992, 1994a).

Continued medical involvement in assisted conception has expanded medical capacity to intervene effectively in reproductive processes, displacing attention from this fundamental problem to (none the less crucial) questions about the quality of medical activity and the efficacy of the solutions proposed. In a sense, what now essentially justifies medical intervention in matters pertaining to sex and reproduction is the fact that, however unorthodox the methods, they tend to produce the desired result: a pregnancy which hopefully will go to term.[19] This does not, however, deal with the question as to what decisions and actions regarding procreative matters the participants who are arranging and mediating reproductive transactions can (or must) legitimately assume, and what decisions and actions, to the contrary, do not specifically derive from their domain of competence.

Reproductive choices, in those aspects of childbearing over which one does have some measure of control, imply decisions concerning whether or not one wishes to have children and, if so, with whom, when and in what circumstances. Of course, having children is not necessarily the result of a conscious decision-making process: social pressure, interpersonal conflict and personal ambivalence often interfere with complex biological processes not totally under our control, making the final result of our reproductive lives quite different from our original vision. Nevertheless, development of techniques such as contraception, abortion, and now assisted conception has reinforced the idea of reproduction as a project and a consciously controlled process.

Increase in technical control over our reproductive processes, and assisted conception in particular, implies entry into a new type of reproductive relationship, loosely defined as therapeutic, in which some reproductive decisions are in fact being transferred to physicians. These may, at first glance, appear as technical problems: for example, screening a semen provider for disease transmissible through sperm or deciding on whether a particular couple's request for DI is medically justified. In fact, major reproductive choices, about whether or not, with whom, when and in what circumstances, are being made in the light of norms and values proper to the sphere of medical activity. This, however, may not immediately be apparent because, for two centuries now, these norms and values have been progressively making their way into the minds and actions of both lay and medical people, seeking adjustment with those constructed through personal experience of sexuality, (in)fertility and the family.

The social complexity of the network of relationships in DI (from the semen provider through medical mediators to the recipients) opens up an institutional no man's land between medicine and the family where negotiations and decision-making are taking place. All parties are apparently endeavouring to achieve the same goal: the birth of a healthy child.

Difficulties may nevertheless arise from the fact that medical and family participants do not have a similar understanding of the situation that brings them together or of the objectives they are jointly trying to attain. Tension ensues when norms and values from these two worlds eventually clash, as they are brought to bear on a reproductive decision, for which the customary references are those related to sexuality. Questions about how to proceed may thus occasionally elicit different responses from each of the participants. Given the unorthodox therapeutic stance of physicians engaged in what is essentially a reproductive procedure, it may no longer be evident to the participants involved *what the fundamental choices are and who should be making those decisions*.

In particular cases, decision-making may involve weighing the physician's responsibility for the safety and the favourable outcome of a procedure against a provider's or recipient's right to make major reproductive choices affecting his/her personal life. But how does one define 'favourable outcome' when a procedure involves conceiving a child? Is it conception, an on-going pregnancy or the birth of a healthy child? How does one define 'healthy'? Is the physician's competence and responsibility engaged only as far as conception, the immediate goal of the technical procedure, or does his/her act entail responsibility for the state in which the child will be born? If so, to what extent? If not, are there minimum precautions which must nevertheless be taken by any physician enacting a procedure? In fact, what care should be given to immediately existing 'patients': the woman, the provider, the partner? Do the deontological questions raised by a reproductive procedure differ essentially from those raised by traditional therapeutic situations? If so, in what way? Do different definitions of favourable outcome radically affect interpretation of a physician's responsibility? What relative weight, if any, should be given to a physician's responsibility for the outcome of a reproductive procedure, in view of a patient's ethical competence and right to autonomy in making personal reproductive choices and decisions?

Controversy over who should be making fundamental decisions ultimately leads to the question of 'the welfare of the child' quite simply because, in the long run, favourable outcome usually implies, for all the participants involved, a birth. It may even become an issue in itself to determine who, among the different protagonists, may be considered to have the best interests of the yet unborn child in mind (Bateman Novaes and Salem 1998). There is really no objective answer to this question, when deciding on a course of action; at most, the number of persons and institutions who express concern in such a conflict suggests the wide variety of perspectives that can be brought to bear on this question. A response will therefore depend on the answer given by each society to another crucial question:

how should rights and responsibilities for fundamental decisions be distributed and/or shared?

The overall social consequences of reproductive choices and decisions (birth rate, sex ratio, over-population, etc.) are fundamental political issues; no society is therefore indifferent as to the way in which the question of reproductive rights and responsibilities is raised or to the manner in which it will be discussed and ultimately decided. Physicians, as representatives of a critical social institution with an ever-increasing scope of professional competence, may, more often than not, be called upon to assume such responsibility, by elected representatives of society and even by 'patients' themselves, especially if our expectations grow regarding their technical competence. This would however reinforce the present medicalisation of what are essentially moral and social issues. Examining more closely the questions raised by greater decisional leverage for those who seek and for those who contribute to medical assistance with conception, and exploring possible consequences for individual persons, for family relationships, for medical practice and more generally for society at large, may be a way of finally dealing straightforwardly with the issues raised by the dissociation of fertility from sexual intercourse.

NOTES

I would like to thank Gwen Terrenoire for agreeing to read the final draft of this chapter at such short notice, and for her incisive comments which helped me substantially in revising and completing it.

1. In some countries the diaphragm and even the turkey baster have been used as instruments for those who prefer to 'do it themselves'
2. Anthropologists and historians studying attitudes to infertility in other societies have shown that men are held responsible for a woman's sterility only when they are considered impotent (Héritier 1984; Jacquart and Thomasset 1985). Rejection of responsibility for problems with a couple's fertility quite obviously reflects concern, even today, with sexual potency, in that capacity to transfer semen to the woman's body for conception remains one of the factors (but not the only factor) affecting fertility (Novaes 1994a).
3. The idea of imitating natural processes, at the basis of eighteenth-century experimentation and found quite specifically in the comments on Spallanzani's work by his contemporaries such as Senebier (da Silva 1991) is still used today as a way of expressing what some perceive as the only justified use of assisted conception. One example is a recent decision by a French court, turning down a request by a woman undergoing *in vitro* fertilisation for transfer of frozen embryos after the death of her husband: his death dissolves the couple, and thus the basis for medical intervention, 'imitating natural procreation' (Jugement du 11 mai 1993 du Tribunal de Grande Instance de Toulouse). See Bateman Novaes and Salem (1998).
4. The first recorded use of artificial insemination by a physician, Dr John Hunter,

in England, involved the wife of a clothes merchant suffering from hypospadias, resulting in retrograde ejaculation (Home 1799).

5. This information was also provided in a conversation with Professor Georges David (June 1995). He has recently examined the contents of several letters sealed and deposited at the French Academy of Medicine with the intent of registering a discovery or innovation without publicly revealing its nature ('plis cachetés'). If the letters are not opened at the physician's request during his/her lifetime (usually as a means of contesting someone else's claim to precedence in innovating or discovering a procedure) and if there are no objections from descendants, these letters are opened after 100 years have elapsed for an evaluation of their contents. Several physicians during the 1840s deposited such letters, believing they had each been the first to use assisted insemination. It is both interesting that physicians did not wish publicly to claim first use of this procedure and that they often used it to solve problems which were not explicitly related to a physical incapacity to procreate (David 1987).

6. Despite current use of the word 'donor' to designate the man who anonymously provides semen for insemination, I will opt for the term 'semen provider' used by Ken Daniels, as often as the context and syntax allow for use of the term. It has the advantage of bringing out more clearly certain aspects of semen provision unrelated to gift-giving. This is also important because semen provision is not always solicited as a donation.

7. These were, until quite recently, current practices (Curie-Cohen et al. 1979).

8. Because of the secrecy surrounding donor insemination, very little can be known precisely about the informal arrangements that took place between the participants in this procedure. Basic elements characterising these situations can nevertheless be reconstituted from interview material with physicians, who began their careers at a time when instrumental insemination was still a quasi-clandestine practice (Novaes 1994a).

9. Banks may often be involved in other activities, such as storing the semen of men who are to undergo vasectomy or medical treatment known to have a negative effect on spermatogenesis (radio and chemotherapy, for example). Some semen banks, adjacent to gynecological-obstetrical hospital or clinical services, also extended their practice to the storage of frozen embryos, when *in vitro* fertilisation became a current practice. The data and arguments in the following four paragraphs are based on a field study of French semen banks, conducted between 1986–1990. (Novaes 1986, 1994a).

10. In 1973, Sherman makes what, in retrospect, are many prescient and awesome statements about the future applications of frozen human semen through such research. He mentions not only benefits for those affected by infertility, but also cryopreservation to ensure that 'the reproductive effectiveness of a husband or desirable donor can be extended indefinitely'; to contribute to 'population control', meaning not only the 'reduction of the number of births in our world's population explosion but also the genetic improvement of the population', in particular through H. J. Müller's concept of 'germinal choice' (Müller 1961, 1963; also see note 15); to 'minimise or obviate the potential genetic dangers of man's exposure to radiation on earth and in space and help control mutations of this sort in the population'; to preserve 'spermatogonia and oogonia by freezing or freeze-drying, to cultivate these gonia on demand,

to select sex and other genetic characteristics, and finally to realise *in vitro* fertilisation and development': all this while awaiting 'some degree of chemical control of heredity [which] is on the horizon of man's biologic destiny' (Sherman 1973: 405–6). He was nevertheless forced to conclude that 'the conditions in medical practice, especially the requisite demand for clinical application of frozen stored semen and the economic balance of time and effort, still were not conducive to favourable development', and that 'low temperature research on human spermatozoa had not been a serious concern of the cryobiologist' (Sherman 1973: 399).

11. As is the case in France: the new 'bioethics law' (Loi du 29 juillet 1994) stipulates that the principle of anonymity applies to the donations of all body elements, that donor and recipient must thus not know each other, and that no identifying information may be revealed, unless there is a 'therapeutic necessity' to do so (for example a kidney transplant between compatible relatives) (Art. L 666–5). As for couples who resort to donor insemination, written consent must be given before a judge or a 'notaire' (legal official specialised in contract law), but under 'conditions which guarantee secrecy' (Art. 311–20). The British Human Fertilisation and Embryology Act (1990) is not as restrictive and makes limited provision (in its Section 31) for access to genetic information by those born from assisted conception procedures. This provision apparently does not allow for access to the identity of the donor (Morgan and Lee 1991).

12. An infertile husband may eventually disown a child born by donor insemination: a turn of events which some physicians find unacceptable. In France, the first such case went to court in Nice, in 1976, and since that time, French physicians involved in semen banking have often been among the first to demand legislation regulating the practice of and the problems raised by donor insemination (Novaes 1991, 1992).

13. In France, this deontological position on the part of physicians has become an article in recent regulation concerning assisted conception (loi du 29 juillet de 1994). Sweden's law, quite exceptional for its more flexible provisions related to the identity of the semen provider, correspondingly restricts donor insemination to married couples (Ewerlöf 1985). British law has fewer restrictive provisions, but allows the physician to refuse a procedure to a woman if s/he deems that the welfare of the child may be at stake, including the child's needs for a father (Section 13.5). This stipulation was recently put to test by a court case (R. v Ethical Committee of St Mary's Hospital of Manchester *ex parte* Harriot 1988) and confirmed (Morgan and Lee 1991: 29, 194).

14. For example, the recent development of a new experimental fertilisation technique, intracytoplasmic sperm injection (ICSI), can serve as an alternative to donor insemination if male infertility is due to a low sperm count. In fact, only one sperm is needed for injection into the woman's egg, but this requires her to be subjected to an *in vitro* fertilisation procedure.

15. The use of donor insemination for eugenic purposes is a proposal that has in fact already been made in the past: Hermann J. Müller (1890–1967), an American biologist and geneticist, Nobel prize winner of physiology and medicine in 1946, and sympathetic to socialist ideas, felt that the voluntary use of insemination with specially selected donors could be a means of favouring socio-economic development through the reduction of the 'genetic load' of

mutations in the human gene pool (Müller 1961: 1963; also see note 10 above). Müller later realised that his proposal raised many questions, both from a genetic and a social point of view. None the less, his idea was taken up by Robert K. Graham, in founding the Repository for Germinal Choice (better known as the Nobel Prize winners' semen bank). The screening of semen providers for the possible transmission of genetically determined disease or malformations thus remains a particularly sensitive issue (Novaes 1994a, 1994b)

16. Although there may appear to be some medical advantages to asking married men with healthy children to be donors, the fact that a donor is fertile and has healthy children does not mean that his semen will be fertile in the conditions of donor insemination. He might also have a recessive hereditary condition which his own partner does not have, but which a future recipient might (Jalbert *et al.* 1989; Novaes 1994a, 1994b).

17. Ken Daniels (1987, 1988) has made similar observations in favour of exploring with the donor the possible consequences of semen donation on his relationship with his partner, in a cultural context where the partner's consent is not required.

18. Only the semen provider's rhesus factor can eventually be considered as an element chosen strictly on medical terms (to avoid tissue incompatibility of the pregnant woman's and the foetus' Rh factor, leading to the breakdown of the foetus' red blood cells, usually during a second pregnancy). Even the choice based on blood type has, as its underlying logic, that it should not be possible to reveal through blood typing that the child was engendered by another man than the one legally recognised as his/her father.

19. This statement does not ignore that there is much discussion about the rates of success of different techniques: this is particularly true in the case of *in vitro* fertilisation. It still remains that, as long as some patients are able to have healthy babies by these techniques, any difficulties in the procedure can always be seen as capable of improvement through research, experimentation and evaluation. We should note, however, that frozen semen for donor insemination is today the preferred option in many countries, when in fact fresh semen is at least twice as effective in terms of results, for reasons related to measures taken to prevent the transmission of disease through sperm. Efficacy as such is therefore not a decisive argument with respect to other considerations.

REFERENCES

Bateman Novaes, S. *see* Novaes, S.
Bateman Novaes, S. and Salem, T. (1998) 'Embedding the embryo'. In Harris, J. and Holm, S. eds., *The future of human reproduction: ethics, choice and regulation.* Oxford: Oxford University Press.
Catholic Church. Congregation for the Doctrine of the Faith (1987) *Instruction on respect for human life in its origin and on the dignity of procreation: replies to certain questions of the day (Donum Vitae).*
Curie-Cohen, M., Luttrel, M. S. and Shapiro, S. (1979) 'Current practice of artificial insemination by donors in the United States'. *The New England Journal of Medicine* 11: 585–90.
Daniels, K. (1987) 'Semen donors in New Zealand: their characteristics and attitudes'. *Clinical Reproduction and Fertility* 5: 177–90.

(1988) 'Artificial insemination using donor semen and the issue of secrecy: the views of donors and recipient couples'. *Social Science and Medicine* 27(4): 377–83.

(1989) 'Semen donors: their motivations and attitudes to their offspring'. *Journal of Reproductive and Infant Psychology* 7: 121–7.

(1994a) 'Assisted reproductive technology policy in New Zealand: needs, rights and responsibilities'. *Public Sector* 17(3): 22–5.

(1994b) 'The Swedish Insemination Act and its impact'. *Australian and New Zealand Journal of Obstetrics and Gynaecology* 34(4): 437–9.

Daniels, K. R., Lewis, G. M., Gillett, W. (1995) 'Telling DI offspring about their conception: the nature of couples' decision-making'. *Social Science and Medicine* 40(9): 1,213–20.

David, G. (1985) 'Don et utilisation du sperme'. In Actes du Colloque *Génétique Procréation et Droit* (1985). Arles: Actes Sud, pp. 203–28.

(1987) 'Lés debuts de l'insémination artificielle au XIX⁰ siècle: à propos de quatre plis cachetés. In La Vie des Sciences, *Comptes rendus de l'Academie des Sciences*, série générale, 5: 449–58.

(1991) 'L'insémination artificielle et le système CECOS'. In CECOS (Fédération Française des Centres d'Etudes et de Conservation des Oeufs et du Sperme Humains), *L'Insémination artificielle*. Paris: Masson, pp. 1–20.

Englert, Y. (1994) 'Artificial insemination with donor semen: particular requests'. *Human Reproduction* 9(11): 1,969–71.

Ewerlöf, G. (1985) 'Artificial insemination – legislation'. *Current Sweden* 329: 1–10.

Finegold, W. J. (1976) *Artificial Insemination*, 2nd edn. With a forward by A. F. Guttmacher. Springfield, IL: Charles C. Thomas.

Frankel, M. (1973) *The public policy dimensions of artificial insemination and human semen cryobanking*. Washington DC, George Washington University (Monograph 18 – Program of Policy Studies in Science and Technology).

Giordan, A. dir. (1987) *Histoire de la biologie*, Volume 2. Paris: Technique et Documentation – Lavoisier.

Gregoire, A. T. and Mayer, R. C. (1965) 'The impregnators'. *Fertility and Sterility* 16(1): 130–4.

Haimes, E. (1990) 'Recreating the family? Policy considerations relating to the "New" reproductive technologies'. In M. McNeil, I. Varcoe, S. Yearley, eds., *The new reproductive technologies*. London: Macmillan Press, pp. 154–72.

(1992) 'Gamete donation and the social management of genetic origins'. In M. Stacey, ed., *Changing human reproduction*. London: Sage Publications, pp. 119–47.

Hamberger, L. (1986) 'Artificial insemination by donor (AID) in Sweden'. *Human Reproduction* 1(1): 49.

Handelsman, D. J., Dunn, S. M., Conway, A. J., Boylan, L. M., and Jansen, R. P. S. (1985) 'Psychological and attitudinal profiles in donors for artificial insemination'. *Fertility and Sterility* 43(1): 95–101.

Héritier, F. (1984) 'Stérilité, aridité, sécheresse: quelques invariants de la pensée symbolique'. In M. Augé and C. Herzlich, eds., *Le Sens du mal: anthropologie, histoire, sociologie de la maladie*. Montreux: Editions des Archives Contemporaines, 1984.

Home, E. (1799) 'An account of the dissection of an hermaphrodite dog. To which are prefixed some observations of hermaphrodites in general'. *Philosophical Transactions of London* 89: 485–96.

Jacquart, D. and Thomasset, C. (1985) *Sexualité et savoir médical au moyen age*. Paris: Presses Universitaires de France.

Jacobs, S. (1993) 'Smart sperm'. *Boston Globe*, 12 September, 1: p. 39.

Jalbert, P., Leonard, C., Selva, J., and David, G. (1989) 'Genetic aspects of artificial insemination with donor semen: the French CECOS Federation guidelines'. *American Journal of Medical Genetics* 33: 269–75.

John Paul II (1995) Encyclical *Evangelium vitae*.

Kunstmann, J.-M. (1979) *L'insémination artificielle avec sperme de conjoint: analyse de résultats dans une série de 128*, thèse pour le doctorat en médecine, Université Pierre et Marie Curie (Paris 6), Faculté de Médecine Pitié-Salpétrière.

Mayr, E. (1982) *The growth of biological thought: diversity, evolution and inheritance*. Cambridge, MA: The Bellknap Press of Harvard University Press.

Morgan, D. and Lee, R. E. (1991) *Blackstone's guide to the Human Fertilisation and Embryology Act 1990: abortion and embryo research, the new law*. London: Blackstone Press Ltd.

Müller, H. J. (1961). 'Human evolution by voluntary choice of germ plasm'. *Science* 134: 643–9.

(1963) 'Genetic progress by voluntarily conducted germinal choice'. In G. Wolstenholme, ed., *Man and His Future*. Boston: Little, pp. 247–62.

Novaes, S. (1986) 'Semen banking and artificial insemination by donor in France: social and medical discourse'. *International Journal of Technology Assessment in Health Care* 2(2): 219–29.

(1989) 'Giving, receiving, repaying: gamete donors and donor policies in reproductive medicine'. *International Journal for Technology Assessment in Health Care* 5(4): 639–57.

(1991) 'Vide juridique: notion-écran en l'absence de repères sociaux? L'encadrement législatif de la procréation artificielle'. In F. Chazel and J. Commaille (sous la direction de), *Normes juridiques et régulation sociale*. Paris: Librairie Générale de Droit et de Jurisprudence, pp. 233–41.

(1992) 'Ethique et débat public: de la responsabilité médicale en matière de procréation assistée'. In A. Cottereau and P. Ladrière, eds., *Pouvoir et légitimité: figures de l'espace public*. Paris: Editions EHESS (Coll. Raisons pratiques, vol. 3), pp. 155–76.

(1994a) *Les passeurs de gamètes*. Nancy: Presses Universitaires de Nancy.

(1994b) 'Beyond consensus about principles: decision-making by a genetics advisory board in reproductive medicine'. In Kurt Bayertz, ed., *The concept of moral consensus: the case of technological interventions into human reproduction*. Dordrecht: Kluwer Academic Publishers, pp. 207–21.

Purdie, A., Peek, J. C., Irwin, R., Ellis, J., Graham, F. M., and Fisher, P. R. (1992) 'Identifiable semen donors – attitudes of donors and recipient couples'. *New Zealand Medical Journal* 105: 27–8.

Seligman, Susan V. (1995) 'Au coeur d'une banque de sperme: de l'ampoule de semence à la recherche d'un peu de père'. *L'Actualité* (Montréal), reproduced in *Courrier International* 241 (15–25 juin): 24.

Shenfield, F. (1994) 'Particular requests in DI: comments on the medical duty of care and the welfare of the child'. *Human Reproduction* 9(11): 1,976–7.

Sherman, J. K. (1964) 'Research on frozen human semen: past, present, and future'. *Fertility and Sterility* 15(4): 485–99.

(1973) 'Synopsis of the use of frozen semen since 1964: state of the art of human semen banking'. *Fertility and Sterility* 24(5): 397–412.

da Silva, S. M. (1991) 'L'imaginaire scientifique de la reproduction artificielle au XVIIIᵉ siècle. Mythomania genitalis'. In S. Novaes, ed., *Biomédecine et devenir de la personne*. Paris: Editions du Seuil, pp. 89–130.

Snowden, R. and Mitchell, G. D. (1981) *The artificial family: a consideration of artificial insemination by donor*. London: Allen and Unwin.

Thouret, M. A. (1803) *Application sur l'espèce humaine des expériences faites par Spallanzani sur quelques animaux, relativement à la fécondation artificielle des femmes ou résultats d'une expérience qui prouve que l'on peut créer des enfants avec le concours des deux sexes mais sans leur approche*. Paris: Thourens.

US Congress, Office of Technology Assessment (1988). *Artificial insemination: practice in the United States: summary of a 1987 survey – background paper*. OTA-BP-BA-48 (Washington DC: US Government Printing Office).

7   Regulation of donor insemination

Robert Blank

Introduction

This chapter shifts attention to the public policy context of DI and to the question of what role, if any, governments ought to play in regulating fertility and infertility services. After briefly discussing the wide range of approaches for organising, monitoring, and regulating DI services, it explicitly contrasts the professional model with public regulatory models. The role of the public regarding technological applications in a democracy is analysed. It is argued that while the issues raised by DI make it a matter of public concern and that some form of public accountability is essential, there are dangers to excessive public control of DI services. Attention then turns to a description of current regulatory strategies both within and across nations. The UK Human Fertilisation and Embryology Authority is examined in detail as a model for a state licensing authority. The chapter concludes by proposing a regulatory approach that combines elements from both professional and public models.

Justifying intervention and regulation in the practice of donor insemination

Although DI itself is a simple technique, it is critical to note that it does not stand alone in practice but rather must be seen in combination with other more intrusive and costly assisted reproductive technology (ART) techniques. It is only one of many services provided by most fertility clinics and, thus, will generally be included with them in any guidelines or regulations. Even on its own, however, DI raises broad questions over societal goals and priorities which include:

(i) what level of technological intervention is appropriate for dealing with infertility?

(ii) who should determine whether DI should be applied in a particular case?

(iii) should DI be equally available to all persons?

(iv) what impact will widespread use of DI have on children, women, men, families, minority groups, and society in general?

These broad questions on social goals raise specific policy issues surrounding DI which centre on access, protection of the parties involved, and the use of public funds. First, who should have access to DI? Although this issue recently has focused on policies that exclude single, fertile women, access is also affected by the level of overall funding available and its distribution across public and private facilities, the geographical distribution of services, the length of waiting lists in the public and the private sectors, and access to information about DI services. Even in the absence of categorical barriers to access, socio-economic inequities often translate into inequitable access to DI services. To what extent should the government intervene to assure equity?

Secondly, because the deliberate goal of DI is to produce a child, the state has an obligation to protect the interests and needs of the children conceived by this means. To the extent that these 'products' of DI are affected by the conduct of the services provided, they are a matter of public concern. Key elements for the protection of children are adequate donor screening programmes for genetic diseases, AIDS and other communicable diseases; counselling of prospective parents; and clarification of the legal status of DI children.

A third set of public issues centres on protecting the consumers of DI services. Even when DI is a public, non-profit service, questions of safety, efficacy, and informed consent are crucial. The fact that DI services increasingly are commercial enterprises in many countries raises further concern over the marketing of DI. In a competitive marketplace, consumer protection against false or exaggerated claims by entrepreneurs is considered a state function. Whether implemented through licensing regulations, contracts, or civil torts, the government has a duty to protect its citizens. 'Let the buyer beware' is no longer operative in most Western countries. Therefore, as fertility services increasingly move toward a for-profit setting or even a 'pay-as-you go' system, the argument that they remain free from government regulation is weakened. Moreover, the vast proportion of DI practices that are legitimate have a stake in protecting themselves and should welcome consumer protection policies.

Finally, there is the issue of public funding of DI services. Although it is not likely that the costs of DI will be borne fully by governments, should public funding be provided for couples or single women who lack the necessary resources in order to minimise socioeconomic discrepancies in access? Should such funding be through provision of DI in public facilities or through reimbursement to private facilities? Who is eligible for public support for DI and for what purposes? As DI increasingly is used in combination with other forms of ART including sperm separation techniques for sex preselection (Office of Technology Assessment, 1988), the question of funding becomes more controversial especially in light of restrained health care budgets.

The issues surrounding access and funding become more complicated when DI is used for non-medical purposes. Examples are the use of DI for fertile single or lesbian women, or for purposes of sex or characteristic preselection. These and other potential applications based on preference of individuals, not infertility, raise critical concerns over the allocation of health care resources for non health-related purposes. Although it might make sense to limit access to medical techniques and services to persons with clear medical indications, drawing lines would be difficult and enforcement would be virtually impossible. Furthermore, decisions such as the recent one by the New Zealand Human Rights Commission which, in effect, ruled that limiting access to DI services to infertile couples was in violation of anti-discrimination legislation opens the door to a wide range of non-medically indicated applications that serve the desires of protected groups. At some stage, clarification of acceptable uses of scarce health care resources must take place within the broader social context, thus requiring government action.

Governments have the power to regulate ART should they choose to do so. Although to date few governments have done so, other areas of health care are highly regulated in most Western democracies. This regulation can come in the form of licensing, funding restrictions, or direct agency control. In some cases, the authority to regulate ART technologies can be derived from a new interpretation of existing statutory authority (for instance, DI could be included in adoption statutes), but in other cases it might require a newly framed policy. Although any governmental action ultimately will be judged against the rights of the consumers and the providers of DI services, the formal capacity of governments to regulate its use are extensive. A critical issue then is the extent to which regulation of DI should be a matter of public concern. Before turning to a discussion of the role of the public, regulatory options for DI are discussed.

Regulatory options for donor insemination

Figure 7.1 illustrates the regulatory options available for DI ranging from individual practice on the one hand to national legislation on the other. Given the complexity of fertility services, it is likely that any activity will involve some combination of these mechanisms. Until the mid twentieth century, the practice of medicine was largely treated as a private matter between the health professional and the patient. Professional ethics and

----

Individual	Programme	Professional	Commissions,	Government	Licensing	Legislation
Clinician	Guidelines	Association	Committees,	Guidelines	Regulations	
		Guidelines	Task Forces			

Figure 7.1 Regulatory mechanisms: a continuum

standards of practice provided a guide to clinician discretion, but overall the individual physician held considerable autonomy. Moreover, reproduction being an activity where state interference can easily lead to infringement of individual rights and abuse of state power, makes a private contract model reinforced by confidentiality and personal autonomy intuitively attractive.

However, while some degree of clinical judgement by individual practitioners is essential in order to deal with specific contingencies that arise in each case, general programme guidelines are established to clarify DI protocol for selection, procedures, and access. These criteria might be set by hospital boards of management or ethics committees, but most often they are developed by the staffs of the programmes themselves (Daniels and Taylor 1993).

Although some observers favour this decentralised private regulatory approach where each programme retains autonomy, professional association guidelines offer consistency across programmes and more accountable protections for all involved parties. This mechanism shifts professional control from individual practitioners and programmes to state, national or international associations, but is nevertheless acceptable to many clinicians for the protections it offers those who adhere to the guidelines and because it might serve to preempt government intrusion. This form of self-regulatory model in theory has defined medical accountability through which violators of the guidelines face professional sanctions.

Although professional standards promulgated by such private organisations (for example, see American Fertility Society 1988, 1990) are very valuable and provide some control over the practice of DI, they lack the legal authority to ensure compliance. Instead of force of law, association guidelines rely on creditation privileges and ethical sanctions. Without state requirements such as the UK licensing authority, there is, however, little to stop the establishment of non-accredited or non-sanctioned fertility clinics or DI services from operating on their own outside the jurisdiction of the professional association: 'Lack of adherence to professional standards is a serious problem in donor insemination. It may be that guidelines require further publicity, directed especially toward DI practitioners who are not fertility society members.' (Achilles 1992: 7). Although lack of compliance with voluntary guidelines by nonmember businesses carries some risk, in the emerging highly lucrative commercial fertility industry, such guidelines might, in themselves, not be a strong enough form of self-enforcement or policing of such activities. This has led to calls for some force of law at the least to ensure that such standards apply to all DI services.

As noted in earlier chapters, DI brings with it an array of philosophical, moral, psychological, social and legal issues which elevate it to the public agenda. There is increasing evidence that many fertility specialists themselves would welcome guidance on these issues (Bonnicksen and Blank 1988). Although they largely reject regulations that would interfere with professional autonomy when exercising clinical judgement, 'they would prefer to operate within a set of clearly specified guidelines determined by a publicly appointed and/or approved body' (Daniels and Taylor 1993: 1474). Similarly, a survey of IVF directors found support for government policies that help clarify IVF practice but oppose restrictive policies (Bonnicksen and Blank 1988).

As a result of the broader issues surrounding assisted conception many commissions, committees, task forces or other ad hoc bodies have been established to investigate ART and advise governments as to what, if any, action to take. Knoppers and Le Bris (1991) found that over 100 reports existed by 1991 on the ethical and legal issues associated with ART. Although some of these reports were non-governmental, most were government initiated. Despite the continued proliferation of such reports there has been little action (statutory, regulatory, or guideline) by governments. It is unclear whether the incongruity between the volume of government-commissioned reports and the paucity of government action in response to them reflects the political use of such *ad hoc* bodies as deflective mechanisms by elected officials or an acknowledgement that the issues raised by ART are too complex or politically sensitive for decisive action.

The limits of public regulatory models

Despite factors that appear to justify a public role in regulating DI services, public choice in medical matters remains problematic. Bonnicksen, for instance, argues that public action is 'unlikely, premature, and unwise in many areas of biomedicine' (1992: 54). Rapidly changing technologies and social values raise prospects of instant obsolescence of any law no matter how carefully framed (Walters 1987). Legislation, then, risks freezing technology in place and is unlikely to offer the flexibility needed to adapt to new applications. Furthermore, the moral underpinning of the debate over reproductive technologies and their tie to abortion means that legislation is likely to be made on the basis of emotions rather than dispassionate, rational choice. There is no guarantee that government involvement will be objective nor helpful in resolving the problems discussed above.

Societal issues

↑

Bioethical deliberation

↑

Identification of clinical issues

↑

Clinic rules

↑

Professional guidelines

↑

Private policy

Figure 7.2 Progression of processes in private policy. *Source:* Bonnicksen (1992: 54)

Attempts to fit medical decision making into models used for other areas of public policy also fail to account for several unique features of medicine. First, as noted earlier, traditionally the conduct of medical decision making has been based on professional judgements made without governmental intervention and monitored primarily by medical standards of care. Government involvement in the 1970s largely reinforced this tradition by granting the medical community accountability through the establishment of institutional review boards and ethics committees. A second special feature of medical decision making is its focus on the human body. As such it is protected by constitutionally based liberties and the common law principle of self-determination. Governmental intervention in the physician–patient relationship necessarily involves substantive decisions about medical care that can 'threaten individual liberty and medical privacy' (Bonnicksen 1992: 54). All governments have at their disposal a broad range of powers to intervene in matters of public health. Although courts in most democracies traditionally have been hesitant to intervene in medical decisions concerning individual patients, increasingly they are becoming embroiled in birth and death decisions.

In order to avoid the dangers inherent in applying public choice models to medical decision making, Bonnicksen argues that the focus of medical decisions should remain outside the public sector. Although there is a need for standard and systematic rule making in medicine, this is better served by a private policy model which 'views regularized rules and procedures in the medical setting as the desired end of biomedical decision-making' (Bonnicksen 1992: 54). To this end, figure 7.2 illustrates the progression of processes that culminate in private policy or 'rules developed in the private sector . . . regarded as obligatory by those who practice' (Bonnicksen 1992: 61). Such policy, then, is manifested by professional society guidelines that somehow are binding on all practitioners in a given field. Unfortunately, Bonnicksen does not explain how this will be accomplished without some type of universal accreditation licensing authority.

Public control in a democracy

While the debate at the practical level turns on whether a public or a private regulatory model is the most effective and feasible approach, at the conceptual level debate centres on the role of the public in a democracy. Should there be a public role in decision making regarding the use of public funds for ART services including DI? It is useful to examine this controversy as a conflict between two democratic models, the technocratic elite model and the egalitarian model.

The technocratic elite model emphasises the democratic ends rather than the means of making the decision. Technocracy is ruled by technically competent professionals and assumes that modern problems require a degree of knowledge beyond the technical capacity of both citizens and their elected representatives. Experts alone have the interest and knowledge necessary to make informed decisions on these complex and largely technical issues. Moreover, in medical areas the critical role of professionals trained to make clinical decisions makes public control unfeasible. In fact, according to this model, to expand public control is to invite trouble because resulting decisions are bound to be uninformed and simplistic.

In contrast, proponents of broadened public control emphasise the importance of the means of making democratic decisions. They argue that the public is as qualified as experts to make policy decisions on issues that are as much social and moral as they are technical. The extensive social and legal consequences of specific technological applications warrant close public scrutiny. Although there is a tendency for some supporters of public control to assume that the entire public ought to be involved in policy making, it is more reasonable to define the effective public as composed of more or less specialised attentive publics and the elected representatives. Although public control does not exclude a role for experts, ultimately the decisions are made by the public through the government. (See chapter by Edwards in this volume.)

There is a need for conceptual clarification of the applicability of public control based on the distinction between making technical decisions requiring medical expertise and establishing broad social priorities as to the goals of medicine. While the first dimension depends on technical competence, the second depends on moral competence, which is not monopolised by experts. Figure 7.3 illustrates the interaction of this specialised–generalised continuum with the competing models of democracy.

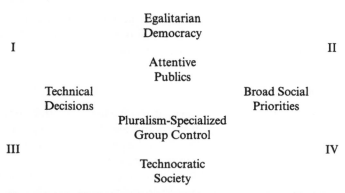

Figure 7.3 Public role in making policy. *Source:* Blank (1990: 198)

The weakest case for egalitarian democracy is in quadrant I. Continued low levels of scientific and technological literacy exhibited by the populace (Miller 1989) make it problematic that many citizens are able or willing to develop a familiarity with the technical aspects of medical technology. Similarly, technocrats have no valid claim to monopolise decision making in quadrants II and IV, which are dependent on moral, not technical, competence. Expertise in a technical area does not ensure, and in some cases might even obscure, attentiveness to the social implications of technology. The kind of specialised knowledge experts have is not adequate in itself to deal with the unique ethical value dimensions of these issues. Although technical experts must be included in the debate over social priorities, and, in fact, might take the lead in a public debate, extensive public involvement is most critical here: the closer we approach full participation, the better for democracy.

Realistically, then, quadrants II and III represent the focus in the debate over public participation. Although the size and quality of the attentive public should be widened at all levels, as we move from the establishment of binding social priorities toward making highly technical decisions, more and more specialised groups take on greater importance. As we shift from deciding what the right ends of social policy ought to be, to how to carry out these goals, the scope of participation, by necessity, narrows. The extent to which DI regulations are a public or a private responsibility, then, depends on whether they are seen as being solely technical in nature or representing broader social issues.

There is, of course, no guarantee that democratising DI policy making would lead to enlightened decisions or resolve the issues discussed here. However, by opening up the regulatory process, it is likely that resulting policies would be perceived more favourably by the public and viewed as more accountable to the public. Although this public debate would focus on the broader social issues surrounding DI, the result would be to legitimise the entire package of regulations. Furthermore, 'If a wide variety of views and opinions were taken into account there would be more likelihood of arriving at decisions that reflected a balance between competing perspectives' (Daniels and Taylor 1993: 1479). Although the advantages of public participation and a governmental role in DI policy might in the end be largely symbolic, proponents of all but a strict technocratic model of democracy would see this enterprise as valuable.

Current regulatory context: nations and states

The public mechanisms used to cope with the ethical, legal, and political issues raised by reproductive technologies vary widely across countries and states. Primarily, these activities represent a combination of legislation, administrative regulations, reports of commissions or other *ad hoc* bodies, and court opinions. Legislation, both federal and state, has been adopted in some countries to deal with particular techniques or applications. In some cases, the appropriate legislation is new, while in other cases existing legislation such as family law, adoption law, and criminal codes have been adapted, extended, or interpreted to apply. In parliamentary systems, government White Papers or Consultation Papers, which often serve as the basis for future bills, continue to serve as guidelines until legislation is passed. Other bases of control are public health and licensing regulations, issues papers, and departmental reports.

In most jurisdictions, the initiative for regulations and legislation has come from the reports of various forms of national commissions, legislative standing committees, and departmental committees (e.g., the Warnock Committee Britain (1984), the Waller Committee in Australia and most recently the Baird Commission in Canada (1993)). In some cases, extensive hearings and public dialogue have accompanied the actions of these bodies. In other countries, the initiative has come from national medical associations, medical societies, or legal societies. Some of these attempts at self-regulation have resulted in placing the issues on the public agenda. Alternately, in several cases these professional guidelines have become *de facto* public policy. Finally, in the absence of enabling legislation or regulations, the courts in a few countries continue to be the most visible source of policy making in response to reproductive technologies.

At least thirty-five countries have either legislation, regulations, or guidelines concerning the practice of DI. Table 7.1 illustrates the major issues surrounding DI which have been addressed by governmental action and shows what mode of control is presently in use in each country. The table

Table 7.1. *Summary of DI regulations by country*

Country	Mode of control	DI child legitimate	Heterosexual couples only	Licensed facilities only	Screening donors	Records required	Payment to donor
Australia	States	yes	yes	varies	yes	yes	expenses only
Austria	Legislation	yes	yes			yes	no
Belgium	Legislation	yes					
Brazil	Prohibit DI						
Bulgaria	Legislation	yes	yes		yes		
Canada	States/commission	yes	generally	yes	yes	yes	expenses only
Czechoslovakia	Legislation	yes	yes		yes		
Denmark	Legislation	yes	priority	yes			
Egypt	Prohibit DI						
Finland	Practice						
France	Commission	yes	yes	yes	yes	yes	no
Germany	Report	yes		yes	yes	yes	no
Greece	Legislation	yes					
Hungary	Legislation	yes			yes		
Iceland	Commission						
India	Practice						
Ireland	Professional guidelines		yes				
Israel	Regulations	yes	yes	yes	yes		
Italy	Regulations		married only	yes	yes	yes	
Japan	Professional guidelines	yes				yes	yes
Libya	Prohibit DI						
Mexico	Practice						
Netherlands	Council	yes			yes		travel only

New Zealand	Commission	yes	singles		yes	
Norway	Legislation	yes	yes	yes		
Poland	Courts	yes				no
Portugal	Regulations			yes		
South Africa	Regulations		yes	yes	yes	
Spain	Commission	yes	singles	yes	yes	
Sweden	Legislation	yes	yes	yes	yes	
Switzerland	Commission	yes		yes	yes	
United Kingdom	Legislation	yes	no	yes	yes	yes
United States	States	yes	generally	yes	varies	yes

should be interpreted with caution because continuous changes quickly date any such effort. Furthermore, it represents only a summary description of a more complicated situation where there exists considerable variation within some countries, especially federal systems such as Australia, Canada, and the United States. About half of these countries have legislation or regulations regarding DI, while the remainder depend primarily on commission reports or professional guidelines.

Is donor insemination allowed? The first policy decision, and one which shapes the need for further action, is whether the practice of DI is allowed. Only three of these countries prohibit the practice of DI under all circumstances. The 1957 Code of Medical Rules in Brazil bans DI, although it permits artificial insemination by husband (AIH) if both spouses consent to the procedure. In Egypt too, AIH is allowed but DI is not. The most extreme negative response to DI is that of Libya where it is a criminal offence. The person who arranges an insemination or actually inseminates a woman, the woman herself, and her husband if he consents to the procedure, are all subject to imprisonment under Libya's criminal code (Articles 304A and 304B). Unlike Brazil and Egypt, it is unclear whether AIH is permitted under Libyan law.

Legitimacy of donor insemination children. In those countries which allow the practice of DI, a major concern centres on the legal status of the children born through DI. Although the wording varies, most of the countries that have adopted laws on DI specify that, if the husband consents to the procedure, the resulting child is considered his legitimate offspring. A 1987 Belgian law, for instance, states that the child of DI with consent of the husband is legitimate and that the consenting husband cannot challenge paternity (Office of Technology Assessment 1988). Likewise, a Greek statute (1983) states that the husband who has consented to his wife's undergoing DI cannot disavow paternity of the resulting child. The Family Law of Czechoslovakia (1982) states that the consenting husband may not contest paternity if the child is born six to ten months after DI. Similarly, the Swedish AI Law (1984) requires written consent of the woman's husband or cohabitant, who as a result is regarded as the legal father. Bulgaria's Family Code (Article 31) also states that the consenting husband cannot later contest paternity (Office of Technology Assessment 1988).

In those countries without legislation, most committees and courts have recommended that laws be enacted to legitimize the children of DI. A report of a Canadian Advisory Committee on Storage and Utilization of Human Sperm (1981) urged that the child be considered the legitimate offspring of the woman and her consenting husband. Provincial reports reinforced this recommendation. Similarly, directives of the Council of Medical Research in Norway (1983) state that DI children should be considered legitimate. In Austria, a study recommended that DI be used only if the husband or partner is sterile and all parties give informed consent (Ministry of Sciences and Research 1986). If so, paternity cannot be contested after the fact. In Poland, a 1984 Supreme Court decision denied the consenting husband's challenge of paternity following DI (Office of Technology Assessment 1988). In Germany, in the absence of legislation, two conflicting court decisions have left the status of DI children unclear, although the later decision gave the consenting husband no right to contest the legitimacy and paternity of the resulting child (Mutke, Bleichrodt, and Theiler 1986).

There is developing consensus among those countries that allow DI that written consent of the husband or partner of the woman undergoing DI is essential if the child's legal status is to be assured. In many countries, however, this does not guarantee that a lawsuit over custody will never be filed, but consent makes it unlikely such a suit will be successful. In South Africa (1986), permission of the donor's wife is also required and, in France (1988), the sperm donor must be married and of proven fertility.

Access to donor insemination services. Although access to DI is dependent on socioeconomic, geographic, and funding factors, issues over barriers to single and lesbian women's access are likely to escalate. Increasingly, practices that exclude singles and lesbian couples will be challenged on constitutional or discriminatory grounds. A 1994 ruling by the New Zealand Human Rights Commission which found such practices in violation of the Human Rights Act illustrates the broader social issues over access (Christchurch Press, 24 July 1994: 5).

While there is some evidence of change, most countries that have addressed this issue limit DI access to married couples or heterosexual couples in a stable relationship. Sometimes, as in the case of France, which limits DI to stable couples but only if the male is sterile or has a genetic disorder, other restrictions are present. The 1985 Santosuosso Report in Italy proposed that DI be limited to married couples and available only when adoption is not granted within six months of application (Mori 1987). Under Sweden's DI law (1984), a physician must ascertain the couple's psychosocial circumstances and verify that they are both medically fit. Only married women or women cohabiting with a male can use DI services because 'a child needs both a mother and a father' (Achilles 1992: 23).

A special parliamentary commission for the study of Human In Vitro Fertilization and Artificial Insemination (1986) in Spain recommended that single women be able to receive donor sperm for insemination if they can demonstrate the capability to provide an adequate home. Ontario's Law Reform Commission report on artificial reproduction (1985) would restrict access to stable single women and to stable men and stable women in stable

marital or non-marital unions. Although Denmark (1987) does not prohibit single women from its DI programmes, it has a policy of giving priority to married and cohabiting women. Israel (1987) limits DI to married or
long-term *de facto* heterosexual couples. Moreover, in Australia, legislation
in Victoria (1987) limits access to married couples, while South Australia
(1987) restricts access to married or *de facto* couples if their relationship has
lasted for at least five years. (See chapters by Lasker and Novaes in this
volume.)

Access to DI can also be circumscribed by legal constraints on where it
may be performed. Such restrictions, which are found in approximately ten
countries, also enable administrators to monitor and regulate the practice
more easily. The two general approaches are to require that DI services be
performed either in public facilities or by licensed practitioners. In Norway,
for instance, a 1987 law demands that DI be performed only at designated
hospitals, with special authorisation from the Ministry of Social Affairs,
and under the direction of trained specialists. Similarly, a 1984 Swedish law
mandates that DI be performed in general hospitals and under the super-
vision of obstetricians/gynaecologists.

DI in Germany is practised in special infertility centres only, while, in
Portugal, DI is available in publicly created centres or by private doctors
who have been specially licensed by the Ministry of Health. Likewise, under
Ministry of Health regulations in Israel, DI may be carried out only by a
licensed obstetrician or gynaecologist after thorough examination of both
the husband and wife. Finally, South African regulations limit the practice
of DI to physicians who are registered and approved by the Director
General of the Department of National Health and Population
Development (1986).

Regulating donor insemination services. In addition to potential state
control over what agencies or persons can perform it, public health regulations can be initiated to specify how they perform it. About one-half of the
countries that have addressed the issue of DI require screening of semen
providers: for sexually transmitted diseases (eleven countries), for genetic
disorders (twelve countries), or both (nine countries).[1] Also, because of the
threat of the transmission of HIV through DI, other countries are taking
steps towards screening. In South Africa, recipients are screened for the
same conditions as the provider to ensure they are suited for DI 'biologically, physically, socially, and mentally' (Office of Technology Assessment
1988: 341). They must also be advised by the physician of the psychological
and legal risks of DI. Most countries have not adopted clear regulations
concerning the screening of providers despite the clear threat of the transmission of disease through donor sperm. Often where professional guidelines are considered adequate, state action is not sought.

In the United States a few states have taken statutory actions, although most have not. In 1981, Oregon passed a law that prohibited persons who knowingly have a genetic or venereal disease from being semen providers (Ore. Rev. Stat. sec. 109. 239). Idaho, too, makes it a violation of the Code (secs. 34–5401 to 39–5408, 1985) for a man who knowingly has a genetic or venereal disease to be a semen provider. Ohio requires, in addition to a full physical examination and genetic history, genetic screening of all DI providers. Only New Mexico limits the number of offspring per provider, even though this is recommended practice. Furthermore, twenty-one states require that DI be performed only by a licensed physician, presumably to assure at least some provider screening. The Georgia DI statute (Ga.Code Ann. sec. 74–101.1, 1973), for instance, provides that licensed physicians and surgeons are the only persons authorized to perform DI upon any female. Any other person who attempts or actually administers or performs DI is guilty of a felony, with threat of punishment by imprisonment for not less than one year and not more than five years.

Although payment for sperm providers is routine in the United States and allowable in the United Kingdom and Japan, most countries that have addressed the issue reject payment. The Ontario Commission report recommends that providers be paid reasonable expenses as do the state committee reports in Australia. The Health Council of the Netherlands allows travel expenses only. In contrast, Belgium, France and Portugal do not permit any compensation, while Germany has outlawed the sale or purchase of human gametes. Moreover, in some countries, such as New Zealand, the issue of payment for human sperm or ova has not arisen because of a strong tradition of voluntarism.

Another area of concern in regulation of DI services centres on the question of whether there should be limits on the number of times the semen of a particular provider can be used in order to reduce the chance of consanguinity. To date, at least eight countries have accepted the principle of setting limits although only a few have actually specified the number of children allowed (South Africa, five; Spain, six; Austria, ten; and Germany, one or ten, depending on which report recommendations are accepted). Because of its small population and, thus, heightened concern over this issue, Iceland imports all its sperm from Denmark.

Maintaining and accessing records. Most of the countries which have dealt in-depth with DI (through legislation, regulation, or comprehensive reports) require detailed record-keeping, although they differ as to what should be done with the information. Although most of the countries that require extensive records about the donor state that complete anonymity is essential, the Benda (1985) report in Germany concludes that the child conceived through DI should have access to this record when he or she turns sixteen years of age. The 1984 AI law in Sweden requires that information about the sperm provider be kept on special hospital records for at least seventy years. At the age of eighteen, the child has a right to learn the identity of his/her biological father. In effect, the law equates DI with adoption, giving the provider a socially recognized position, but with no rights. Furthermore, the public welfare committee is duty bound to assist the child in retrieving this information. Although the parents are not obliged to disclose to the child the use of DI in his or her conception, the National Board of Health and Welfare encourages them to do so.

Except for Austria, which has adopted the Swedish law as a model for its own, few other countries appear inclined to take steps in the direction of Sweden. The Australian Medical Procedures Act (1988) requires a central registry of certain non-identifying and identifying information about providers and recipients. Non-identifying information is to be accessible to all parties and identifying information is to be made available upon obtaining written permission of the person inquired about. Under Israeli regulations, strict records of the semen provider are kept, but the identity of the provider remains confidential. A select committee in Spain and most state and provincial committees in Australia and Canada have recommended central registries of all donor inseminations, with access to non-identifying information by the child at age eighteen.

The UK Human Fertilisation and Embryology Authority. One regulatory model which has considerable promise is the Human Fertilisation and Embryology Act passed by the UK Parliament in 1990. This Act . . . 'introduces statutory control of a new form of clinical practice; it brings to the forefront of attention questions as to the provision of and payment for assisted conception services' (Morgan and Lee 1991: 23). The Act is the culmination of almost a decade of debate in Britain that emerged from the Warnock Committee (1984) recommendations and replaces the interim statutory licensing authority. Under the Act a new authority, the Human Fertilisation and Embryology Authority (HFEA), was established to design a national system to regulate certain practices involved in the treatment of infertility and research on human embryos. Its jurisdiction includes DI but not AIH.

Of direct relevance to DI, the HFEA is required to operate a licensing system for all centres that store gametes or offer treatment which involves the use of donated gametes. A Licensing and Fees Committee is empowered to ensure that no prohibited activities take place and that no activities for which licences are required are undertaken without said licence. Centres seeking a licence must provide information about staffing, facilities, patient information leaflets, consent forms, record forms, operating procedures, and charges. Inspection teams visit each site. An inspection fee is charged, but the largest part of the Authority's income will be raised through annual fees charged to centres based on the numbers of treatment cycles performed in the year prior to application (Daniels 1992: 4). Treatment and storage licences may be issued only for a maximum of five years, after which re-application must be made.

The HFEA will also maintain a central registry of all covered treatments, all children born as a result of treatment, and all semen providers. Among its other statutory duties are publication of a Code of Practice, guidance to centres on how to carry out licensed activities, and advice to providers and prospective providers and to persons seeking treatment. The object of the Code of Practice goes beyond securing the safety and efficacy of treatment and research practices to areas of practice which raise fundamental ethical and social questions, with special emphasis on the right of people who are or may be infertile to proper consideration of their request for treatment and concern for the welfare of children. It is expected that licensed centres comply with the Code in terms of staffing, assessment of providers, information for patients and providers, welfare of the children, consent, counselling and use of gametes unless they can show good reason for not doing so in a particular case (Daniels 1992: 5). The Code of Practice is to be regularly reviewed to ensure continued relevance to changing circumstances.

Conclusions

This review of current governmental activities in regulating DI demonstrates that with a few notable exceptions, there is a lack of systematic and coherent societal guidance for the practice of DI. There is a clear need for consistency that at present is lacking. While professional association guidelines in many countries are valuable as far as they go, because they lack the force of law, compliance is often poor. DI policy in most countries is the product of a patchwork and often haphazard combination of programme and professional guidelines, committee reports, court rulings and in some cases statutory regulations. Moreover, often the statutory requirements represent new interpretations of existing laws poorly fitted to DI. This divergent and potentially conflicting combination of private and public actions results in ambiguous policy.

Although in some jurisdictions this fragmented regulatory framework appears to be adequate for protecting all the parties involved, extensions of DI into non-clinical areas promise to test this framework. Moreover, most current provisions focus on the technical aspects of DI, thus leaving the broader social, psychological, and ethical issues unresolved. As stated earlier, these issues should be addressed through a societal-wide dialogue extending beyond the medical community. It ought to be interdisciplinary and open to all interested segments of the public.

Within the context of the discussion of decision-making models in a democracy the regulation of DI must include both technical and broader societal components. One approach would be to allow appropriate professional associations to establish specific standards for the technical aspects of DI. These recommended standards would then be open to a public consultative process and eventually codified into regulations that are binding on all practitioners and programmes offering DI services. Concurrent with this policy-making process would be a public dialogue on the goals of ART technologies including DI and on social priorities in offering such services. This debate would include consideration of questions of access; protection of the parties to DI including children; and public funding and allocation priorities.

The UK HFEA might serve as a useful model for similar regulatory approaches in other countries. Although the licensing authority strategy must be adapted to the political structures of each country, it has the potential of offering an optimal mixture of private input and public control if the technical aspects are derived from professional guidelines. Despite the need to monitor closely the impacts of the HFEA on DI and to ensure that it is flexible enough to respond to changing technological and social applications, the concept is sound. This licensing model of regulation has the advantage of public control and programme accountability that is lacking under a private, professionally controlled model.

The task of establishing a consistent national policy for DI services is made all the more difficult in federal systems where health policy and licensing are largely under the jurisdiction of the separate states or provinces. It is no surprise that the HFEA emerged first in the UK and not in the United States, Australia, or Canada. Although national commissions have recommended guidelines in federal systems, the fragmentation of power has made adoption of national standards in those countries problematic. This decentralisation can also create conflict between national professional association guidelines and state licensing and regulatory policies.

The options introduced earlier provide a rich and varied array of mechanisms for regulating DI. Although I believe licensing regulations through legislation offer the most effective means of assuring compliance to standards of practice and providing consistency, the evidence presented here suggests that regulation of DI in most countries will not take such form in the foreseeable future. This in part reflects limitations on the public model as suggested by Bonnicksen's (1992) critique and puts more pressure to develop adequate private policy. In most countries, however, it appears that DI will continue to be practised within a haphazard and often ambiguous regulatory environment represented by a mix of private and public mechanisms.

NOTE

1. Countries that require screening for sexually transmitted diseases include Australia, Canada, France, Hungary, Israel, Italy, Netherlands, New Zealand, South Africa, Spain and the United Kingdom, as well as parts of the United States. Countries that require screening of semen providers for genetic disorders include Australia, Bulgaria, Canada, Czechoslovakia, France, Hungary, Israel, Netherlands, South Africa, Spain, Switzerland, the United Kingdom and parts of the United States.

REFERENCES

Achilles, Rona (1992) *Donor insemination: an overview.* Ottawa: Royal Commission on New Reproductive Technologies.

American Fertility Society (1988) 'Revised new guidelines for the use of semen donor insemination'. *Fertility and Sterility* 49(2): 211.

(1990) 'New guidelines for the use of semen donor insemination: 1990'. *Fertility and Sterility* 53(3): Supplement 1.

Baird, Patricia (1993) *Proceed with care: final report of the Royal Commission on New Reproductive Technologies.* Ottawa: Minister of Government Sources.

Blank, Robert H. (1990) *Regulating reproduction.* New York: Columbia University Press.

Bonnicksen, Andrea L. (1992) 'Human embryos and genetic testing: a private policy model'. *Politics and the Life Sciences* 11(1): 53–62.

Bonnicksen, Andrea L. and Blank, Robert H. (1988) 'The government and in vitro fertilization (IVF): views of IVF directors'. *Fertility and Sterility* 49: 396–8.

Brazil (1957) Code of Medical Rules, Article 53.

Canada Advisory Committee to the Minister of National Health and Welfare (1981) *Storage and utilization of human sperm.* Ottawa: Minister of Government Services.

Canadian Fertility and Andrology Society (1988) *Guidelines for therapeutic donor insemination.* Montreal: CFAS.

Christchurch Press (1994) 'Fertility Ban on Singles Illegal'. 24 July.

Czechoslovakia (1982) Family Law, Article 52-2.

Daniels, Ken (1992) 'The UK Human Fertilisation and Embryology Authority – one year on'. *The Fertility Society of Australia Newsletter* 25: 4–5.

Daniels, Ken and Taylor, Karyn (1993) 'Formulating selection policies for assisted reproduction'. *Social Science and Medicine* 37(12): 1,473–80.

Denmark (1987) Law No. 53 on Establishment of an Ethical Council and Regulation of Certain Forms of Biomedical Research.

France (1988) Act on Artificial Insemination [Law No. 88–1138, 20 December 1988].

Georgia Code (1973) Annotated Section 74–101.1. Norcross, GA: Harrison Company.

Greece (1983) Civil Code [Article 1471/2-2, Law 1329].

Idaho Code (1985) Sections 34–5401 to 34–5408. Indianapolis: Bobbs-Merill.

Israel (1987) The Public Health Regulations of 1987.

Knoppers, B. M. and Le Bris, S. (1991) 'Recent advances in medically assisted conception: legal, ethical and social issues'. *American Journal of Law and Medicine* 17: 329–61.

Miller, Jon D. (1989) Personal communication on status of National Scientific Literacy Study.

Ministry of Sciences and Research (1986) *The Fundamental Aspects of Genetics and Reproductive Biology*. Vienna, Austria: Ministry of Sciences and Research.

Morgan, Derek and Lee, Robert G. (1991) *Blackstone's guide to the Human Fertilisation and Embryology Act 1990*. London: Blackstone Press Ltd.

Mori, Maurizio (1987) 'Italy: pluralism takes root'. *Hastings Center Report* 17(3): 34–6.

Mutke, H. G., Bleichrodt, W. H. and Theiler, R. (1986) 'Legal aspects of artificial insemination by donor in the Federal Republic of Germany: the first judgments in 1982 and 1985'. *Human Reproduction* 1: 420.

National Bioethics Consultative Committee (1991) *Access to reproductive technology. Final report for the Australian Health Ministers' Conference*, Canberra.

Norway (1983) Council of Medical Research. *Directives in ethical matters for artificial insemination and in vitro fertilisation*.

Norway (1987) Act relating to artificial procreation [Law No. 68, 12 June 1987].

Office of Technology Assessment (1988) *Artificial insemination: practice in the United States: summary of a 1987 survey*. Washington, DC: US Government Printing Office.

    (1988) *Infertility: medical and social choices*. Washington, DC: US Government Printing Office.

Ontario (1985) *Report on human artificial reproduction and related matters*. Toronto: Law Reform Commission.

Oregon Revised Statutes (1981) Section 109: 239. Salem, Oregon: Statute Revision Council.

South Africa, Department of National Health and Population Development (1986) 'Regulations regarding the artificial insemination of persons'. *Government Gazette* 10,283: 28–35.

South Australia (1987) South Australian Parliament. Legislative Council. *Report of the Select Committee of the Legislative Council on artificial insemination by donor, in vitro fertilisation and related matters in South Australia*. Adelaide: Government Printer.

Spain (1986) Special Commission for the study of in vitro fertilization and artificial insemination, 'Informe', *Boletin Oficial de las Cortes Generales* 166: AD 38–1 (21 April).

Sweden (1984) Act on insemination [Law No. 1140, 20 December 1984].

Victoria (1987) Infertility (Medical Procedures) Act of 1984, amended 1987.

Walters, Le Roy (1987) 'Ethics and new reproductive technologies'. *Hastings Center Report* 17: 35–95.

Warnock, M. (1984) *Report of the Committee of Inquiry into human fertilisation and embryology*. London: HMSO.

Jeanette Edwards

An anthropological perspective

Developments and innovations in assisted conception have raised questions that go beyond the practical and pragmatic application of the techniques themselves. In Britain, for example, attention has focused on, amongst other things, whether or not women should be allowed to donate ova to their sisters, whether maternal surrogacy arrangements should be allowed, or, in the case of DI whether sperm providers should be, and remain, anonymous. From a social anthropological perspective, such concerns reveal a culture's understanding of the way in which significant social relationships are created and maintained. Stories about conception and the ways in which people perceive themselves to be related, as well as the forms that such relationships take, come under the rubric of kinship; and the demarcation of kinship and its study has been central in the development of social anthropology.[1]

This chapter draws on anthropological research in a town in the north of England, which for present purposes I call Alltown.[2] I returned to Alltown, a place where I had previously carried out residential fieldwork, in order to investigate residents' ideas about new reproductive technologies.[3] In the process of this research, I was constantly 'passed on' to residents who were perceived to have different kinds of knowledge about creating and maintaining family relationships. Hence, women said I ought to speak to men, or to other women who were perhaps younger or older, or to other women who had smaller or larger families – to people, in other words, who were perceived to have a different experience of kinship. In making sense of assisted conception, the Alltown people with whom I spoke, drew on cultural notions of procreation and of what constitutes relatedness; they drew on their expertise of kinship. Thus when they thought about substituting the ova of sisters, they focused on the implications such a procedure might have for the relationships involved: for the way in which each woman would be related to the child, to each other, and to their respective partners. They made sense of the implications, then, not through what they know about the techniques and philosophies of reproductive medicine but through the social relationships it has the potential of creating and affecting (Edwards 1992, 1993). The relatively simple techniques of DI, compared to the medically intrusive procedures of *in vitro* fertilisation (IVF), do not make the social relationships involved any less complex.

This chapter will focus on the way in which people in Alltown, at the beginning of the 1990s, explored limits to the possibilities presented by the medical assistance of conception. A concern over limits has been a common feature in the media coverage of different aspects and techniques. It has also been apparent in the deliberations of service providers and in the views of those commissioned to advise on social policy. The Warnock Report on Human Fertilisation and Embryology, commissioned by the British government in 1982, was explicit in this respect: 'There must be *some* barriers that are not to be crossed, *some* limits fixed, beyond which people must not be allowed to go' (Warnock 1985: 2, original emphasis). The report notes that evidence received by the Committee of Inquiry was as diverse as the opinions of Committee members themselves, but what all had in common was the idea that there ought to be '*some principles or other* to govern the development and use of the new techniques' (1985: 2, original emphasis).

Limits are explored and set at particular historical moments. Ideas about where boundaries should lie are informed both by cultural pasts and by the trajectory of developments. For example, Verena Stolcke writes that the German Benda Report rejected DI 'in the interest of the child's psychic well-being' (1988: 12–13). The same report also addressed a concern that doctors might use eugenic criteria to select appropriate semen providers. It is not far-fetched to assume that the Benda Report's caution about the use of donated semen is informed as much by a historical knowledge of the eugenic policies of the Third Reich, as contemporary ideas about a child's psychological well being. Such concerns appear less evident in the ideals of the Repository for Germinal Choice which, when launched in the USA in 1971, collected sperm exclusively from Nobel prize winners (Kevles 1985), moved on to include non-prize winning scientists and today requires its semen providers to pass an intelligence test (Kevles 1985; Littlewood 1995).[4] Attitudes towards the range of assisted conception techniques are inevitably embedded in, and influenced by, historical trajectories and current political thought. Robert Blank's chapter in this collection discussed the way in which legally sanctioned limits differ between countries.

In this chapter, I argue that contestation over limits is not simply a matter of disagreement between different interest groups, which might have been predicted, nor does it merely indicate different opinions or attitudes of individuals within particular interest groups, which is inevitable, but that it is inherent in the way in which people explore the implications in a cultural context. Drawing on anthropological fieldwork in Britain, I argue that views on assisted conception are ambivalent. And that ambivalence stems from cultural ideas about the way in which persons are reproduced and related.[5] From this perspective, ambivalence is not a prerogative of 'lay' persons but is also mobilised in the views of 'experts'[6]. This leads to a consideration of the notion of 'public opinion'.

I argue in this chapter that delimitation of something called 'public opinion' obscures the process whereby social actors explore the implications of assisted conception in a cultural context. That there is a commitment, in much of the debate over the ethics and techniques of assisted conception to the notion of 'public opinion' is clear. In January 1994 for example, the British media focused their attention on research being carried out into the possibility of using ova from aborted foetuses and cadavers. The resulting furore led more than one scientist to acknowledge that 'the public' were not quite ready to condone the use of eggs from such sources. However, such comments hint that although 'the public' were not yet 'ready' for such procedures, they would eventually come round to the idea. This assumption rests on the premise that people think the way they do because of ignorance or lack of knowledge, and that given information (of the right kind) they will eventually change their opinion.[7] It also rests on the premise that new ideas, by the nature of their novelty, cause anxiety at first, but eventually people become accustomed to them. It is in this context that the notion of 'public opinion' is often evoked, as if it were an entity, uniform and bounded, able to be tapped and then swayed. In these kind of formulations there appears to be a close association between 'public opinion' and 'ordinary people': both are perceived to have neither expertise in the topic at hand nor a vested interest.

It is to the credit of the Warnock Report that for the most part it avoids reference to 'public opinion'. It reiterates forcefully and clearly that there is no consensus on assisted conception, but rather a 'range of views within society'. It is revealing, however, to look at the way in which the Warnock Report represents the diversity of evidence it received. The names of some of the individuals and of all the organisations that submitted evidence to the Committee are provided. For the most part, the list comprises names of interest groups, organisations and institutions, and of the individual experts who provided oral evidence. In addition, the report notes that the Committee received 695 letters and submissions from 'the public' (1985: 101): a category that appears to include all those who wrote neither as professionals nor as members of voluntary or statutory organisations. The Report shows a further commitment to the notion of 'the public' (1985: 52) in its idioms of, for example, 'the public at large' (1985: 1), and 'public . . .

sentiment' (1985: xiv, original emphasis); it also addresses 'public concern' (1985: 75), and identifies former 'public ignorance' (1985: 8), current 'public anxiety' (1985: 74) and changes in 'public attitudes' (1985: 74). 'The public', conceived of as a body (out there, beyond the committee) is ever-present. The report also allows for the idea that some opinions are less well-formed than others, and that new ideas require time to be taken on board. An example of this is Wendy Greengross and David Davies' dissent from the prevailing view that legislation ought to be introduced to prevent surrogacy arrangements on the grounds that 'public opinion is not yet fully formed on the question of surrogacy' (Warnock 1985: 89). Thus the suggestion is promoted that, in time, views will crystallise and opinions form.

We might conclude from the Report that the Committee took into consideration both 'expert' and 'lay' opinions and, although there was widespread agreement on the need for boundaries, there was little agreement as to where to place them. From an anthropological perspective, however, it is difficult to sustain a dichotomy between 'lay' and 'expert' opinion. Both members of the laity and of professions are cultural beings and consequently draw on particular cultural ideas to order and make sense of social phenomena of which they need not, necessarily, have direct experience.[8] Both lay persons and experts draw on their own personal experiences, and their cultural expertise, to make sense of new social phenomena.[9] The views of, for example, 'ordinary people' (the public) and 'philosophers' (experts) may resonate in ways which are not immediately obvious when their membership of an interest group (that is, 'philosophers' or 'ordinary people') is being emphasised. From this perspective, lay and expert understandings might be regarded as folk models (Strathern 1992b) which rely on implicit cultural assumptions about the way in which persons and relationships are reproduced. I want to suggest that by identifying a 'public', with its attendant notion of 'public opinion', the complexity with which *all* social actors make sense of ART is obscured.

In the remainder of this chapter, and drawing on material from Alltown, I explore several aspects of assisted conception that intrigued many people with whom I spoke; each is marked by contradiction and ambivalence and, in exploring the contradictions, my aim is to indicate the difficulty of identifying such a thing as 'public opinion'. I have attempted so far to make explicit the way in which, from an anthropological perspective, the concept of kinship might be mobilised to analyse understandings of assisted conception. In the final section, and in the light of the data presented, I address the question 'why kinship?' But first a brief introduction to Alltown is necessary, and I take that opportunity to present an example of ambivalence that, at first glance, has little to do with assisted conception; namely, the way in which the idiom of the 'tight knit community' is used in Alltown to portray both negative and positive images of the town and its people. I then explore ambivalence in the context of assisted conception. I do so by looking, in turn, at residents' perceptions of the dangers of secrecy, the nature of gametes, the advantages and disadvantages of knowing the source of semen, and ideas about selfishness. I intend to provide the reader with a sense of the context in which such ideas emerge in conversation. While these topics are delimited for analytical purposes, they are, in fact, intertwined and implicated in each other; they constitute cultural understandings of the reproduction of persons and relatedness that are wider than the specifics of reproductive medicine.

Alltown

Alltown has a population of 15,000 people, and lies north of the Greater Manchester conurbation. It grew with the development of the textile indus-try and by the middle of the nineteenth century was a busy and industrious milltown, attracting labouring families from rural areas of England and Ireland. Alltown is conceptualised as a working class town, evidence for which is found in its industrial heritage. However, it would be wrong to assume that this chapter presents the view of only working-class people. The data on which it is based were collected from those who define them-selves as 'Alltown born and bred' and those who think of themselves as 'incomers', and they include those who, in sociological terms, belong to both the working and middle classes. I interviewed women and men who are, amongst other things, houseworkers, factory workers, factory owners, self employed, unemployed, professionals, service providers, students and retired elders. Conversations took place in the privacy of people's homes or in arenas of sociality, such as public houses and local organisations. All the Alltown residents whose views are presented here are white.

Many people with whom I spoke noted that Alltown is distinctive. Residents, both those who think of themselves as born and bred in Alltown and incomers (recent and established), and residents of neighbouring towns as well as a few academics in Manchester, all proffered an opinion about its idiosyncrasies. Dialect, history, the interrelatedness of residents and its climate are some of the things said to differentiate it from other localities. Often it is described in idioms which evoke remoteness: as the 'back and beyond',[10] or as a 'backwater'. Yet Alltown is far from remote, despite what people say. It is true there is no railway station, and the motorway linking the east of the country to the west is four miles away, and the temperature does drop perceptibly as you travel into the town, over the moors. But it is also true that residents shop in the hypermarkets of neighbouring towns;

teenagers alternate between 'lounging' in the town centre and in the shopping malls of neighbouring towns; some residents holiday in Florida, others in Blackpool, and some in both; residents visit relatives in Ireland, or Manchester, or Australia, or South Africa; and many subscribe to Sky or cable television, hire the latest videos from a number of outlets in the town, and follow characters in televised soap-operas with interest. Alltown is no more remote than the urban conurbation from which many present-day residents hail. It is as good an example as any of where 'the public' (were one to be looking for such a body) might be located.

Alltown is often described as a 'tight-knit community'. This has both negative and positive connotations: on the one hand, it is said to be cliquish and parochial, excluding those who do not belong; on the other, it is said to be friendly and welcoming, with residents mutually helping each other. 'Nosy' and 'caring' are flip sides of the same coin, and which side lands depends on the context in which the evaluation is relevant. An often heard comment about the 'tight-knit community' is that 'everybody knows each other'. The 'everybody' that one person knows is not, of course, 'the everybody' that another person knows. But the idioms of interconnectedness which include 'everybody knows each other' and 'the tight-knit community' serve further purposes than the enumeration of relationships. Implicit in these assessments is a contrast with the anonymity and coldness of urban life; Alltown and hence its people are being defined, and are defining themselves, through a comparison with the city and city life. The perceived interconnectedness of residents is said to have developed over time, and has resulted in families knowing other families over several generations, which means, to use an Alltown expression, that 'the skeletons in the cupboard' are known. The idea that 'everybody knows each other', and that for some people that knowledge has a historical depth, and that it concerns family relationships, feeds into ideas about ART. This has implications, as we shall see, not only for the way in which Alltown people perceive the wisdom, or indeed the possibility, of keeping secrets, but also for whether donated semen should come from known or unknown sources.

Secrets and 'do-gooders'

I noted above that Alltown people with whom I spoke drew on what they know of family relationships (often providing concrete examples) in exploring the implications of procedures of which they have no direct experience. In conversations and interviews which focused on techniques of DI, participants often made analogies with adoption. In this and the following sections I provide examples of the context in which analogies are made and implications explored. Here, then, is an outline of one particular occasion that elicited an analogy with adoption which, in turn, led to an exploration of the dangers of secrecy.

A creative writing class meets one afternoon a week in the Unemployed Worker's Centre. During the winter of 1990–1991 it comprised a group of women between the ages of forty and seventy. One of their interests is in autobiography and local history and their teacher is a keen and knowledgeable local historian. The women invited me to attend their classes, initially to talk about my original work in Alltown, and in particular the stories about the past which I had collected. We went on to talk of my current interest in assisted reproductive technologies. The quotations below are taken from the transcripts of our conversations in the class. In exploring different aspects the women often referred to what they knew of Alltown. We talked about whether the use of donated gametes should be kept a secret, and one woman made an analogy with what she perceived to be the dangers of keeping adoption secret. Two women presented examples of people they knew, or knew of, who had found out later in life that they had been adopted as children. The narratives of the women focused on the damage caused by the secret emerging rather than by the fact of adoption. The threat to prior relationships, particularly between the adoptive parents and their child, was emphasised. At the same time, members of the class suggested that the issue was irrelevant in Alltown, as such information would not be kept from children anyway. In the words of a class member: 'In Alltown they'd tell them anyway. They're all straight forward, a cob of coal's a cob of coal'.

Both the idea that secrets are undesirable (because they are impossible to maintain) and the idea that secrets are redundant (because people are straightforward) draw on wider Alltown preoccupations. Comments such as 'everybody knows each other' and all about each other, and the idea that Alltown people are honest and 'down to earth', provide images of what Alltown is not. An implicit contrast is being made with 'the city', or 'the south', or 'London', each symbolising a breakdown of relationships and of trust.

If secrets cannot be kept within 'the tight-knit community', they *ought* not to be kept within the family, as they have a nasty habit of emerging when you least expect them to. Ultimately, the secret (which, when it emerges, becomes a lie) is thought to be more damaging to family relationships than the facts of DI. It is not, necessarily, the use of DI *per se* that is the problem, but the way in which significant social relationships are conducted and maintained. (See chapters by Lasker, Haimes, Daniels and Snowdens in this volume.)

Secrets are undesirable, particularly within families, and they pose a threat to existing relationships as they are bound to emerge when one least expects them to. These ideas and the consequences of origins being revealed inadvertently more often than not explored from the perspective of offspring: either adoptees or children conceived through DI. But this view, like many of those explored in this chapter, has its counter-image, found in common idioms such as 'what you do not know cannot hurt'. A case is made for not revealing genetic origins, which relies on the knowledge that parents are those who nurture children and that relationships are built up through time and effort. There is a danger that revealing the genetic origins of adopted children, or those born through DI, will lead to offspring searching for genetic parents, which will cause anxiety to their families. In this context, it is not only desirable to keep origins secrets, but it is now possible. Except, that is, for the 'social do gooder' who, in this instance, is conceptualised as the expert/professional who thinks it best for offspring to know 'the truth'. The 'social do-gooder' symbolises the danger of disrupting prior and pre-existing relationships, for no good cause: they make explicit a contrast between the 'down to earth' Alltownian and the 'out of touch' city dweller. They have little experience of the town, and their views are perceived to be based on abstractions which are not grounded in the realities of Alltown. Consequently, 'social-do-gooders' plant 'unwanted ideas', irrelevant to the contingencies of Alltown. It is they who make suggestions which, for example, in an analogy with adoption, lead people to go in search of their 'real parents' when their family is at home. The figure of the 'social-do-gooder', out of touch with the reality and pragmatics of family relationships, is used by residents to explore the danger of revealing secrets, albeit from the perspective of parents rather than children. In some contexts, therefore, secrets might be necessary and, in such cases, it is not the nature of Alltown that prevents the keeping of them but the intervention of the 'social do-gooder'.

There are several strands to Alltown views about revealing or keeping secret the facts of adoption, or DI, which appear contradictory when placed next to each other in analysis, as I have done here. The nature of Alltown people, down to earth and pragmatic, is thought to lead them to automatically reveal the truth *and* to see the pragmatic necessity for hiding it. However, such ideas appear contradictory only in analysis; when they are put to work in interaction they are used to address different questions, from different perspectives, for different purposes.

Known and unknown origins

A further area of ambivalence is over the nature and significance of gametes. On the one hand, they are a substance generated by the body, expendable and replaceable: in the words of one Alltown man, sperm is 'just bodily substance'. On the other hand, gametes are part of enduring ties that cannot be severed: 'You would be connected and always would', explained another man, of sperm donation. Analogies are made with blood or with organs; one woman remarked that it would be no different from donating a kidney, but after a while, added that 'it would depend on the bloke'. Some men, she observed, would be too sensitive about their own infertility to want to *know* the semen provider: they would prefer, she suggested, to use semen from anonymous sources. Other women with whom I spoke suggested that genetic ties are more important to men than they are to women.[11]

Section 31 of the British Human Fertilisation and Embryology Act (1990) requires the authority to keep a register containing identifying information about semen providers and children born as a result of donation. This is to allow requests from adults who were conceived with the use of donated gametes, to see whether they are related to intended marriage partners. The danger of incest is evidently at the forefront of legislators' minds. It is also an issue which came up frequently in Alltown.

Different Alltown people argued that names and addresses of semen providers ought to be kept on record. Two interconnected reasons are commonly given for naming the providers of sperm. First, children born through DI ought to be able to trace the donor if they choose to do so in the future; such a view is couched in terms of children being able to trace 'their origins' or 'their roots' and, again, an analogy is made with adoption.[12] Second, if records are kept then incest can be prevented. We return to the notion of incest below, but here I present an example of the way in which roots emerge as significant in conversations about assisted conception, again with a focus on the apparent contradictions.

Mrs D and Mrs L are friends and neighbours, and at the beginning of 1991, they were both in their late twenties and each married with two school-age children. Listen to them talking about roots, first from the perspective of those born through DI, and then from the perspective of semen providers:

MRS D   The same rules as adoption should apply – the child has a right to know. It will want to know 'who do I look like – who is this other person?' – it will be curious to know where its roots are from.
MRS L   The donor should be quite pleased to see the result of donation. Say there are 25 children – that is lovely, great – all the more people you have helped. You have no ties to these people, no obligations. No real moral ties
MRS D   You have done the family as a whole a favour.

This brief extract from the transcript of one of our conversations, highlights a contradiction between roots that axiomatically connect persons (it is therefore merely a case of revealing them) and roots that are only made manifest through interaction and the moral obligations that relationships entail. Mrs L and Mrs D explore connections from the perspective of the semen provider and the child, as well from a wider sets of relationships within which people are located. From the vantage point of the child, connections to providers are enduring, albeit implicit. From the vantage point of the provider, there is no relationship, therefore no ties. And finally the family as a whole are grateful for the numerous relationships created. Views shift according to the perspective taken, but the point is that they are aspects of the same phenomenon. In English kinship constructions, people are connected both through biology and through relationships forged in practice. I return to this point below but, first, one further example of shifting perspectives.

Mr T, a father of two young children, told me that he could '*never* donate sperm' because he would be connected to any ensuing children. Nor does he 'agree with surrogacy' because the woman who gives birth to the child '*has* to be its mother' (his emphasis). He explored, later in the conversation, a hypothetical example of he and his wife requiring fertility services. If they had been infertile, he mused, and had a child with the assistance of a surrogate, but using his sperm and his wife's egg, then the child would, without a doubt, be theirs. If he were to provide sperm, then, he would be axiomatically connected to ensuing children whether a guardian or not. But in the case of surrogacy, his connection is attenuated, as the mother is the woman who gives birth to the child. Unless, that is, it is his sperm and his wife's egg; now the surrogate embodies the relationship between him and his wife. From the perspective of the gestational mother, Mr T identifies an axiomatic connection between her and the child, whereas, from the perspective of the commissioning parents, he identifies an axiomatic connection between the child and its genetic parents.

It is the relationship between the commissioning parents, symbolised in the union of their gametes, which connects them to their child, born of another woman. Roots, therefore, refer not only to genetic connections, or to links with a particular place, but they also embody prior relationships. I provide extracts from a different interview to further exemplify this point. Mrs S is in her late fifties and has two grandchildren. She considers herself to be inextricably connected to her grandchildren and describes herself as 'totally concerned about them as if they were [her] own'. Her son's wife, Paula, was married previously and has two sons, now adults. Mrs S would have liked to have been a grandmother to them, but it was difficult; they were older when she first met them, she explains, and they chose not to call her and her husband 'grandmother' and 'grandfather'. The boys, she explains, had a separate life about which she knew nothing, and a separate family, on their father's side, whom she never knew. 'The little ones', however, she knew from 'day one'; she 'held them at a few hours' and has been involved in their lives from the beginning. For Mrs S, the generosity of her daughter-in-law has a great deal to do with the close relationship she feels she has with her younger grandchildren. She told me: 'Paula included us and let us be part of the kids' lives . . . she has been very generous with them'. Thinking of the implications of her son donating sperm, she wondered whether she would feel related to children conceived using the sperm of her son. After some thought, Mrs S concluded that she would not and explained that she would only feel connected if she *knew* the mother.

For Mrs S, if her son were to provide sperm, she would be unrelated to ensuing children unless there was a relationship between her and the mother of those children. Connectedness, like roots, is not an abstract phenomenon devoid of the relationships they entail. It is possible to be axiomatically connected through genetic links, as Mr T points out: it is also possible for there to be no connection unless there is a relationship.

The idiom of roots came up frequently in discussions about the donation of gametes in Alltown. 'Everybody needs roots', one man told me, 'these children do as well'. Not knowing one's roots means, as another person put it: 'Having no real beginnings, no family and no ancestors'. We might be tempted to read statements about roots as referring to a romantic ideal, which purports that, in the past, before assisted conception, roots were more prolific or deeper. But that assumes we know what roots are. As we have seen, the meaning of roots is neither fixed nor stable. Roots symbolise a continuity between place, person and past. They refer to the prior relationships that constitute a person, but they are not definitive of 'belonging'. As much as children are thought to need to know their roots, they also require love, care and attention in order 'to grow'. They need to be reared in a particular manner in order to 'belong'.

'Keeping it in the family': antipathy and altruism

Thinking of DI, people explored the advantages and disadvantages of knowing semen providers. One of the advantages of using gametes from known sources is that, as mentioned above, children born from such procedures are able 'to know' their origins. This is thought to be of benefit to children psychologically and in the future.[13] Furthermore, if 'origins' can be traced, so too can medical histories which, it is assumed, are useful.[14] What about the possibility, then, of brothers providing semen to brothers? Such a possibility was explored in terms of the advantages and disadvantages of 'keeping it in the family'. For Mr T, substituting the semen of brothers is preferable to using semen from unknown sources: 'the kid will have our ways rather than a complete stranger'. But looked at from another angle the idea of brothers providing sperm to brothers is problematic.

Mrs S is unsure about DI but, she points out, if donated sperm *is* used then donors should not be kin. Family creates other problems. Especially if there was family friction at a later date. Human nature being what it is, you would never be sure when a remark was made that would upset the apple-cart.

Mrs S identifies the unpredictability of family life. She makes explicit what everybody knows, that family relationships are as marked by friction as they are by concord. Thinking of DI the source of sperm and the possibility of brothers providing sperm to brothers, Alltown people draw on cultural understandings of what constitutes a brother. Siblings, in Euro-American kinship ideas, are related through shared biological sub-stance, symbolised in genes or blood. Children inherit equal amounts from their mother and their father, and siblings are characterised by having, in common, inherited substance from the same people. Siblings, then, are per-ceived to share substance. Degrees of relatedness are marked, moreover, by the amount of substance they share. Hence 'half-brothers' or 'step-broth-ers' have one parent in common and are conceptualised as sharing less sub-stance than if they had two parents in common. Shared substance, however, does not cover all aspects of relatedness, and people often remark on the fact that 'half' or 'step' relatives or affines are 'closer' than 'full' relatives. One young Alltown woman told me vehemently that she would 'fight anybody' who suggested her step-brother was not her 'real' brother. Siblings, then, are also related through the quality of their relationship in practice. An adopted child is no less a sibling than a genetically related child. It is thought that siblings ought to interact and have each other's best interest at heart, but it *is* the case that some siblings are 'closer' than others.[15]

In the context of shared substance, brothers are viewed as ideal sperm providers. They are 'made up' of the same substance and therefore 'pass on' the same things to their children. The child of a man is related to that man's parents in the same way as the child of his brother; grandchildren, in terms of relatedness rather than affective ties, are substitutable. Furthermore, substituting the semen of brothers means the provider is 'known' which, as we have seen, is thought to allow for family and medical histories (neces-sary for future psychological and physical well-being) to be retrieved. Siblings from this perspective are ideal providers; they are 'close', both in terms of their genetic constitution, and in the form of their relationship. Closeness, in this context, has positive connotations, but, as we might expect from the discussion thus far, closeness has its downside. Kin may, of course, be *too* close. Brothers cannot provide sperm to sisters, but might to brothers, for example, and fathers may not provide sperm to daughters, but might to sons. Certain possible substitutions are thought automatically to constitute incest; neither a sexual relationship nor the birth of a child is necessary for incest to be implied. Indeed, some people do not differentiate between these possibilities and point out, in the words of one Alltown man, that 'all of this stuff is incestuous'.

Hence, if kin are thought to be the ideal candidates as providers, they are also thought to be the least suitable. Apart from the fact that kin may be too closely related (the gametes of certain categories of kin are not substitutable), kin may be too close literally; proximity itself brings certain problems. Again, Alltown residents draw on, and refer to, what they know of the town and its people when making sense of the implications of brothers providing sperm to brothers. One man argued that men could only receive sperm from their brothers, if their brother lived, for example, in London; if they both lived in Alltown it would be too difficult: 'they'd be bumping into each other every day'. Each encounter would act as a reminder that the child was theirs, in the case of the provider, or not theirs, in the case of the father. Furthermore, it is thought that the use of provided semen from known providers has the potential of setting up a different kind of relationship between the provider and the mother. One is not a parent until one has a child, genetically related or not. The birth of a child has the potential, therefore, for creating a different kind of relationship to the one that would otherwise exist, or indeed to the one that would otherwise not exist, between the mother and the provider. The possibility of setting up a link between a semen provider and a receiving woman jeopardises the relationship between the woman and her partner, thought of predominantly, in this context, as her husband.

The down side, then, to using sperm from known sources, is the potential it has for threatening and damaging pre-existing relationships. The relationship between provider and receiving couple might be placed in jeopardy if the provider perceives there to be a 'special' relationship between himself and the child. It is thought that the father of a child conceived with the aid of his brother, may find it more difficult to appropriate that child as 'his own' if he is constantly reminded that his brother is the genitor. When people think about sisters providing eggs to sisters, a concern is often expressed that the provider might want to 'interfere' in the child's upbringing. The potential for men to 'interfere' in the child rearing practices of another family, was raised on a number of occasions in Alltown, but dismissed as unlikely; this does not diminish the threat that their presence poses to the relationships involved.

The problem of incest not only arises if the gametes of particular categories of kin are combined, it also emerges as significant when semen providers are, and remain, anonymous. A concern commonly aired is that children born from gametes of the same provider will eventually meet up, fall in love and reproduce: committing, albeit unknowingly, incest. The actual statistical risk of that happening may be minute, but the notion of incest acts as a powerful conceptual brake. It places a limit on certain possibilities, and acts to formulate a boundary, beyond which it is danger-ous to venture. Similarly, the actual practice of brothers providing sperm to brothers may not be common, but that is not the point: the way in which people explore the implications of it are informed by their cultural ideas of what constitutes persons and the relationships between them. Ideas about DI reveal as much about cultural notions of relatedness as they do about 'opinions' on certain practices. If this is the case, then we need to look care-fully at what is being carved out as 'public opinion' from the complex ways in which people, as cultural beings, make sense of innovations in human reproduction.

'Virgin births' and selfish desires

During research in Alltown, the so-called 'virgin birth' controversy hit the headlines. The fact that single women were requesting access to DI made the front pages of the tabloid press[16] and the inside pages of the broad-sheets.[17] 'Virgin births' were not an issue which appeared to preoccupy people in Alltown unduly. Indeed, given the tone of media coverage at the time, the general lack of interest shown by residents was striking. One woman, in her seventies, was reminded of her sister when I introduced the subject. She hinted that DI might have been a good thing for her sister, who she described like this:

Joan never bothered about getting married. She looked after her mum and dad. She had good holidays. Never bothered much about men friends. Always been fond of children though – took them on holiday. They were fond of their Auntie Joan. Shame she'd never had any.

In exploring different aspects of assisted conception, Alltown people often referred to the experiences of their own family members.[18] The possibility that people's views or opinions change if, for example, those they love require infertility services, is constantly entertained. In the case of 'virgin births', several commentators noted that those who were critical of lesbians and single women having access to DI, would change their mind if it happened in 'their family'. Alltown people acknowledge that opinions shift; in this context, however, it is not through time or access to 'expert' information but through knowledge of the experiences of those who are related.

Many people with whom I spoke suggested that there was unlikely to be a great demand for 'virgin births'. Mrs D pointed out: 'People don't want millions of kids – they'd probably only do it the once'. She thought maybe it would be confined to 'the upper classes' as only they would consider bringing up children alone. This provoked Mrs L to suggest that perhaps 'the background' of single women should be 'looked into' to make sure they have enough money to provide for a child. Earlier both women had argued vociferously that money should *not* be a criterion for deciding who should be parents. This is an example of the way in which views shift according to the question being addressed, and it is worth, at this point, looking a little closer at the shift between thinking economic factors important and denying their relevance.

Class implications came up frequently in my conversations with Alltown residents. The fact that provision within the National Health Service is limited, while private treatment is readily available, was an issue at the forefront of Alltown concerns. Many people with whom I spoke were adamant that decisions over who should receive treatment, and what kind of treatment, ought not to depend on wealth. Such a view was often linked to ideas about what makes a 'good parent' where, again, the role of money was rejected. Now the kind of relationship between parents and children is emphasised; the quality of relationships is thought to have nothing to do with money. According to one woman, parents require 'a sense of humour', and they 'have to be flexible enough to change their ideals'. And for another, parents have to be able to understand things from a child's point of view; they have to 'come down to the level of the child'.

Running alongside such views is the idea that certain desires and practices stem from having money. Hence only single women who are financially independent would *desire* to bring up a child alone, and therefore request DI services.

Many Alltown people with whom I spoke argued that 'infertile couples' should be helped in whatever ways are available. They point out that social class, money or status should not be the criteria by which decisions as to who should reproduce are reached. They acknowledge what they refer to as the 'heartache' of infertility, and recognise all kinds of pressures, particularly on young women, to have children. They identify a common perception in Alltown that, without children, 'it's not a proper marriage'. And while many women question the idea that women are 'unfulfilled' without children, they also identify a stigma attached to remaining childless. Family, friends, colleagues and neighbours assume that if young, married couples have not conceived a child within two or three years of marriage then there is a 'problem' (Edwards 1995).

It is a knowledge of the kind of pressures on people to have children, as well as limited and rationed health service provision, which inform a view that infertile couples should be helped by whatever means are available. In the words of Mr T: 'everybody should have the right to have children – if

they are about thirty and can't then they should be given the chance . . .
Everybody around here has kids. Couple thirty years old without kids has
never been known.' Mrs D and Mrs L also spoke of the pressure on women
to have children:

MRS D   In a marriage . . . it's a natural thing. Other women push you – they yearn
    for other women to have kids.
INTERVIEWER   Why?
MRS L   Vindictiveness – 'I have so you should'.
MRS D   It's a matter of course – women are labelled as selfish for not wanting kids.

Mrs D was reminded, at this point, of the chat show she had watched that
morning on television, which had focused on the controversy surrounding
'virgin births'. She recalled that in the programme single women had been
labelled selfish for *wanting* children. This provoked her and Mrs L to
explore the inconsistency and sexism in the views put forward on the programme. 'Women are selfish if they have children and selfish if they don't',
remarked Mrs D. They went on to talk of the reasons for people wanting
children and they concluded, *contra* the 'experts' on the programme, that
'*everybody* has a child for selfish reasons' (Edwards 1995).

I have shown how Alltown discussions are marked by ambivalence. This
section has focused on the way in which people argue that decisions over
who should receive treatment should *not* be based on money, and that the
difficulties caused by infertility are such that people should be helped by
whatever means are available. However, running through all the examples I
have discussed is a concern with limits; people express disquiet at certain
techniques and emphasise the need for boundaries and for the excesses of
clinicians and scientists to be curbed.

'Kinship' or 'the family'?

As we have seen, there are as many disadvantages as there are advantages
of 'keeping' DI 'in the family'; some relationships are axiomatically 'too
close' to allow for the substitution of gametes. Brothers are thought to be
competitive, and the inevitable outcome of interaction is conflict. Men, it is
said, need to know their 'own' offspring; they are more likely to care for
'their own' children than those not genetically connected. If the sperm provider is a man's brother, then his presence and continuing relationship
might act as a constant reminder to the recipient that the child is not 'his'.
Such knowledge, it is thought, may compromise the undivided care and
attention a child requires. Parents, as sexual partners, are thought to have
dominant responsibility for child rearing.[19] Hence, when people think
about transferring gametes between sisters, they remark on the danger of

providing sisters 'interfering' in the child's upbringing. Will the woman who provided the egg feel more responsible for the resulting child, than she would as an aunt? Will the brother who provided sperm perceive the resulting child as his? Will the union of his sperm and his sister-in-law's egg (a union that would, without DI, take place through sexual intercourse) imply a bond between them? These questions present the provider as a 'problem' and a potential threat to existing relationships. Erica Haimes (1990) shows convincingly how the call for anonymity of donors in Britain serves to protect the ideal of 'the family'. Hence, if semen providers remain anonymous, the commissioning couple are better able to conform to a dominant notion of 'the family' as a child-rearing unit comprising a heterosexual couple and their biological children. The presence of the provider might act as a reminder that the ideal of the heterosexual couple who are both the biological *and* the social parents has not been met. The data from Alltown confirms this analysis. But, from an anthropological perspective, it also appears that Alltown people are less concerned with an abstract ideal of 'the family' than with the unpredictability of kinship. It is the imperative to preserve significant social relationships in an appropriate manner which appears to drive many Alltown concerns. The fragility of kin relations is as much a concern as genetic continuity, and one does not preclude the other. People identify the potential difficulties of knowing semen providers as well as *not* knowing providers; they also argue that 'infertility' is a terrible thing and *everybody* should have access to fertility services.

Men and women suggest they are more likely to provide gametes to kin than to strangers; whether they do or not is beside the point. Kinship is not a thing to be jettisoned lightly, and obligations and duties stand, whether they are performed or not. The idea that men are less likely to forge bonds through caring may reflect a real state of affairs, where men, in general, take much less responsibility for childcare than women, but this does not preclude the idea that bonds are formed through the practice and practicalities of relationships. While it is thought that men as fathers need to *know* that they are genetically connected to their children, it is also thought that sperm is readily detachable from men. One idea does not preclude the other; they coexist, and are drawn upon to answer different questions and to solve different dilemmas.

Conclusion

It has become almost a truism in social anthropology that making sense of a particular social phenomenon requires an understanding of the social context in which it is embedded. It cannot, in other words, be understood in isolation from cultural understandings and practices with which it is interlinked. As Anthony Cohen forcefully pointed out over a decade ago: 'If you attempt to abstract any piece of social process without full consideration of its cultural context you will derive, at best, only a very partial understanding and, at worst, total misunderstanding' (Cohen 1982: 15). The way in which people make sense of assisted conception needs to be understood in relation to other preoccupations, such as, identity and belonging, the reproduction of class and gender, and the maintenance and creation of social relationships.

Boundaries, the places where limits are set, shift according to the context. The context is immediate. It lies in interaction, and is the question addressed and the perspective taken. Consequently, pinpointing 'public opinion' is not only difficult (opinions shift depending on the question being addressed) but it is misleading. To pinpoint 'public opinion' is to artificially freeze-frame one take of a constantly shifting process. It entails retrieving and fixing one set of views, which are, in fact, but one element in this continuous but not random process.

Alltown people with whom I spoke explored with me the advantages and disadvantages of using sperm from known and unknown sources. They identified advantages and disadvantages of sperm providers being related or anonymous. Family members may be thought of as ideal candidates and arguments are put forward for 'keeping it in the family'. This idea emerges in its contrast with commercial activity. One idea triggers another. Procreation should ideally be kept within the family, which ought to lie outside the market. Alongside such views runs the counter-argument that providers ought to remain anonymous, and the thought of substituting the gametes of kin is enough for the conceptual brake of incest to be applied. These views are not mutually exclusive. They are put forward by the same person, possibly in the same conversation. There is no one answer. There *are* advantages and disadvantages of the two and the issues *can* be addressed from different perspectives and vantage points. In presenting their views from the perspective of the child, or recipient, or donor, Alltown people with whom I spoke about DI draw on their own experiences of family relationships and on their cultural understanding of the reproduction of persons.

People make sense of assisted conception through what they know of Alltown, and through their own experience of kinship. Hence, the issue of 'virgin births' is not something which appeared to preoccupy the people with whom I spoke to the same extent as, for example, the substitution of gametes between kin or surrogacy arrangements. Apart from the idea that it will only involve a few people and, then, those from different classes and, by implication, different places, people also put forward the idea that such a practice is more to do with individuals and, hence, has fewer implications for existing relationships.

The areas of ambivalence I have identified in this chapter generate important questions about the nature of 'public opinion'. It is often assumed that once 'public opinion' is tapped, it can be swayed, or changed, through more information and education. But how accurate is it to think of the way in which people make sense of new possibilities in procreation as opinion? There appears to be neither one public, nor one opinion, and attempts to elicit such a thing must inevitably be an attempt to identify, for a particular purpose, one position from a process of shifting perspectives.

NOTES

I am grateful to Erica Haimes and Ken Daniels for their helpful comments and editorial guidance. My debt to Alltown friends and associates not only remains but grows.

1. The anthropological study of kinship in non-Western societies has often entailed comparison, albeit mostly implicit, with western notions of procreation where biology is highly significant. Biological ties have often been the baseline from which the degree and kind of cultural elaboration is assessed (Gellner 1987). David Schneider (1980, 1984) has argued that the biological is, itself, a symbolic construction; the shared substance of blood or genes symbolises a prior relationship already culturally constructed. For Marilyn Strathern (1992a, 1992b) the biological and the social are inextricably intertwined in western, or what she calls Euro-American, kinship thinking. For discussion of cultural theories of conception see, for example, Malinowski (1982); Leach (1966); Delaney (1986); Franklin (1993, 1997).

2. I carried out residential fieldwork in Alltown between 1987 and 1988 and further research there during the winter of 1990/1991. The name of the town and residents have all been disguised.

3. The study was part of a project (carried out in collaboration with Sarah Franklin, Eric Hirsch, Frances Price and Marilyn Strathern) which aimed to explore how cultural and social implications of assisted conception might be discerned. It was funded by the Economic and Social Research Council (award number R000 232537) and selected findings are published in Edwards *et. al.* 1993.

4. The sperm bank in California is best known for housing sperm of the physicist William Shockley.

5. Although the ethnographic example I draw upon in this chapter is from Britain, it is also an example of Western, or what some scholars refer to as Euro-American kinship thinking (for example, Strathern 1992, 1993, 1994; Rapp 1987; Ginsburg and Rapp 1991).

6. Both Erica Haimes (1993) and Frances Price (1994, 1997) provide interesting examples of this from members of the Warnock Committee and clinicians, respectively. Haimes, for example, analyses the way in which members of the Warnock Committee, on the one hand, make analogies between sperm and egg donation and, on the other, argue that the motives of men who provide semen are different from those of women who provide eggs.

7. I have argued elsewhere (Edwards 1992) that all too often the concern of people to place limits on medical intervention in reproduction is understood by

service providers to stem from ignorance, which in its least offensive disguise translates as lack of information. Much health promotion work has rested on the assumption that all people require is more information, of 'the right kind', in order to change their 'habits' or, to use an overused euphemism, their 'lifestyles'.

8. See, for instance, Franklin (1993) for examples from members of parliament and Haimes (1990, 1993) for examples from members of the Warnock Committee.
9. I have argued elsewhere that Alltown people explore the social implications of assisted conception through their expertise of kinship (Edwards 1992, 1993).
10. 'back and beyond' = back of beyond.
11. Recent research suggests that men in commissioning couples prefer sperm providers to be anonymous and are unlikely to choose a brother as provider (Lessor 1993).
12. Again the stories told of adopted children who attempt to find their 'natural' parents later in life are countered, as mentioned above, by a view that it is 'social do-gooders' who plant such ideas in adoptees.
13. Conversations in Alltown often turned to the implications for children conceived using different techniques. Again people drew on what they know of the place, and often the danger of children being stigmatised was raised. One man remarked:

> [The] fundamental question is, what is the child going to think? Grown-ups are making their plans . . . Not enough consideration on the way the child is going to view this. Too much pissballing about with adults and the science of it and on the relationships of grown-ups, but too little concern about children.

14. A rationale which has little mileage as people also remember that children born through adulterous relationships can not trace their medical histories.
15. For David Schneider (1980, 1986; see also Finch 1989), notions of shared substance are accompanied by 'codes for conduct', which while not necessarily adhered to, nevertheless make explicit the way in which relationships between, for example, siblings *ought* to be conducted. I make the distinction elsewhere between relatedness which is the way in which kin are perceived to be connected, and relationships which emerge from the conduct of the kinship ties (Edwards 1993: 45).
16. For example, *Today, Daily Mail, Daily Mirror*, 11 March 1991.
17. *The Times*, 11 March 1991; *The Independent, The Times, The Daily Telegraph*, 12 March 1991.
18. This was also evident in the debate in the House of Lords (Franklin 1993).
19. A common explanation given by grandparents, not just of course in Alltown, about the special relationship they have with their grandchildren is that, 'at the end of the day they can hand them back'.

REFERENCES

Cohen A. ed. (1982) *Belonging: identity and social organisation in British rural cultures*. Manchester: Manchester University Press.
Delaney, C. (1986) 'The meaning of paternity and the virgin birth debate'. *Man* 21(3): 494–513.

Edwards, J. (1992) 'Local perspectives on new reproductive technologies'. *Anthropology in Action* no. 11 (Spring 1992).

(1993) 'Explicit connections: ethnographic enquiry in north-west England'. In J. Edwards, et. al., *Technologies of procreation: kinship in the age of assisted conception.* Manchester: Manchester University Press.

(1995) 'Imperatives to reproduce: views from north-west England on fertility in the light of infertility'. In R. Dunbar, ed., *Reproductive decisions: biological and anthropological perspectives.* London: Macmillan.

Edwards, J., Hirsch, E., Franklin, S., Price, F., and Strathern, M. (1993) *Technologies of procreation: kinship in the age of assisted conception.* Manchester: Manchester University Press.

Finch, J. (1989) *Family obligations and social change.* Cambridge: Polity.

Franklin, S. (1992) 'Making sense of missed conceptions: anthropological perspectives on unexplained infertility'. In M. Stacey, ed., *Changing human reproduction.* London: Sage.

(1993) 'Making representations: the parliamentary debate on the Human Fertilisation and Embryology Act'. In J. Edwards, E. Hirsch, S. Franklin, F. Price, and M. Strathern, eds. *Technologies of procreation: kinship in the age of assisted conception.* Manchester: Manchester University Press.

(1997) *Embodied progress: a cultural account of assisted conception.* London: Routledge.

Gellner, E. (1987) *The concept of kinship and other essays on anthropological method and explanation.* Oxford: Basil Blackwell.

Ginsburg, F. and Rapp, R. (1991) 'The politics of reproduction'. In *Annual Review of Anthropology* 20: 311–43.

Haimes, E. (1990) 'Recreating the family: policy considerations relating to "new" reproductive technologies'. In M. MacNeil, ed., *The new reproductive technologies.* London: Macmillan.

(1993) 'Issues of gender in gamete donation'. *Social Science and Medicine* 36: 85–93.

Kevles, D. J. (1985) *In the Name of Eugenics.* Harmondsworth: Penguin.

Leach, E. (1966) *Genesis as Myth.* London: Jonathan Cape.

Lessor, R. (1993) 'All in the family: social processes in ovarian egg donation between sisters'. *Sociology of Health and Illness* 15: 393–413.

Littlewood, R. (1995) Mankind Quarterly Again. *Anthropology Today* 11(2): 17–18.

Malinowski, B (1982 [1929]) *The sexual life of savages.* London: Routledge and Kegan Paul.

Price, F. (1994) 'Conceiving relations: egg and sperm donation in assisted procreation'. In D. Pearl and R. Pickford, eds., *Frontiers of family law.* London: Chancery.

(1997) 'Matchmaking in the clinic'. In Clarke, A. and Parsons, E., eds *Culture, kinship and genes.* London: Macmillan.

Rapp, R. (1987) 'Gender politics of Euro-American kinship analysis'. In S. Yanagisako and J. Collier, eds., *Gender and kinship.* Stanford: Stanford University Press.

Schneider, D. M. (1980) *American kinship: a cultural account.* [2nd edition], Chicago: University of Chicago Press.

(1984) *A critique of the study of kinship.* Ann Arbor: University of Michigan Press.

Stanworth, M., ed. (1987) *Reproductive technologies: gender, motherhood and medicine*. Cambridge: Polity.

Stolcke, V. (1988) 'New reproductive technologies – same old fatherhood'. *Critique of Anthropology* 6: 5–32.

Strathern, M. (1992a) *After nature: English kinship in the late twentieth century*. Cambridge: Cambridge University Press.

(1992b) *Reproducing the future: anthropology, kinship and the new reproductive technologies*. Manchester: Manchester University Press.

(1993) 'A question of context'. In J. Edwards, E. Hirsch, S. Franklin, F. Price and M. Strathern, eds., *Technologies of procreation: kinship in the age of assisted conception*. Manchester: Manchester University Press.

(1994) *New certainties for old? The case of enabling technology*. Lancaster: Centre for the Study of Cultural Values.

Warnock, M. (1985) *A question of life: the Warnock report on human fertilisation and embryology*. Oxford: Blackwell.

9 Concluding comments

Erica Haimes and Ken Daniels

As editors we had three aims in preparing this book: to provide the first systematic social science analysis of DI, as the oldest and most widespread technique of assisted conception; to provide an international perspective on DI, given its worldwide status in terms of practice; to make a significant contribution to the widespread debates on practice and policy in the field of DI and to the field of assisted conception more generally. It is clear to us, however, that we have not said everything there is to be said about DI. The purpose of this final chapter, therefore, is not to round off the debates but rather to show how the contributors to this book have advanced the discussion in certain areas and to identify those areas that would still benefit from further investigation and analysis.

Perhaps the first striking feature of this collection is the way in which several contributors have used the 'first story' of DI to orient themselves in terms of the story that they then wish to tell. That first story has given rise to a multiplicity of stories, written and told from a multiplicity of perspectives. It is now very clear that there is no longer one single way of explaining and accounting for DI. All sorts of people have all sorts of things to say about DI, ranging from describing their personal experiences, to expressing views on professional responsibilities, to arguing about ways of ensuring the adequacy of public policy, to speculating about these practices as an ordinary member of the community. We do not mean to diminish their importance by referring to them as stories: rather we want to emphasise that the accounts given, now and in the past, are very much shaped by the authors of those accounts, hence these stories come in all sorts of shapes and sizes and hence they all contribute to the mosaic that is now 'donor insemination'.

However, this notion of authorship and perspective should also remind us that, historically, not everyone has been given an equal opportunity, nor an equal hearing when attempting, to tell their story about DI. We have tried to show in this collection the emergence of some voices that have most frequently been silenced, notably those of the sperm providers and the people conceived. Chapters in this collection suggest that they and others might have much to say that will surprise us but historically their voices have been silenced, not necessarily in the clinic but certainly more widely. From a social science point of view this raises at least two very important questions: first, how has our understanding of DI been shaped by the fact that their voices have not been heard (especially given the point that we make in the Introduction and that is demonstrated in almost every subsequent chapter, that the language and practices of DI are dynamic and are changing all the time) and, second, how has our understanding of DI been shaped by the voices that have been heard and that have been seen as the legitimate representatives of the silenced parties? We cannot know the answers to these questions until those voices are heard more widely and on a wider number of issues. The contributors to this volume have made a start on alerting us to the existence of these other voices and to the fact that there are wider issues surrounding DI but clearly there is still much more that can be done here. For example, what do parties such as the recipients of treatment, the sperm providers and the people conceived have to say about not just their own direct experiences but also about the wider policies and practices that are developing worldwide? And about the fact that they are part of this worldwide development in assisted conception rather than just isolated individuals living out their private lives?

It is clear, if only from the relative lack of attention that DI has received from analysts outside the field of practice, that DI is far from the 'glamorous' side of assisted conception. Whilst IVF received detailed attention from social scientists from its earliest days, DI flourished for a good thirty years before receiving similar attention. Social scientists, who have a tendency to point out the failure of other groups in society to recognise the social implications of certain practices, were themselves very slow in appreciating the social significance of DI. This collection represents the first systematic analysis of DI since Snowden's pioneering work of the late 1970s. Even now this field has received much less attention from certain strands of social science such as feminism than might be expected, and less than IVF and surrogacy for example. Indeed on a broader front, Callahan (1991) has expressed surprise that this practice 'slipped so easily into the mainstream of our society' (1991: 43). He has suggested that a wider public debate still needs to take place, particularly in the United States from where his analysis has emerged. Such a debate would focus on three questions: what can we learn from the medicalisation of DI (see the chapter by Novaes); what should a public debate be about (could it for example cover the question of the public control over the private desire for a family? See the chapters by Blank and by Lasker) and how broad could such a debate be (could it for example question whether DI should be practised at all?).

This raises another set of questions that merits further consideration, but which is largely outside the immediate capabilities of this collection: the extent to which DI is to be considered a unique practice and the extent to which it is to be considered an exemplar or a paradigm for other forms of assisted conception? Certainly DI has to be understood as part of a range of responses to the problems of procreation, but on the other hand, given its prominence in terms of being one of the first responses to the problem of overcoming infertility, it might be considered to have had a particular influence on other later responses. Annas and Elias regard DI as the 'accepted paradigm for all other methods of non-coital reproduction' in terms of the policy responses found in the Warnock Report and the Waller Commission (see Blank's chapter in this collection) but wonder if it is in fact 'an unworkable paradigm' particularly in the way it places the rights of the parents above those of the child (1989: 615). This article by Annas and Elias is a useful example of the temptation to try to consider all the responses to infertility and subfertility in one single way whereas, as the difficulties they experience indicate, this may be an exercise inevitably doomed to failure. That is, it is a mistake to try to achieve consistency or even complete distinction, between all aspects of all forms of assisted conception. If nothing else, the chapters in this collection show the social complexity of even the apparently simple practice of DI. It would appear to be the case that rather than try to place an analytical straitjacket over all the dimensions of all forms of assisted conception, it would be analytically more revealing to consider the parallels and distinctions between various specific dimensions of the different practices. Thus, DI may be a suitable paradigm for considering the rights of the person conceived in all other forms of assisted conception but may be the least suitable comparator when considering the role of the third party across all the different techniques. Again, we do not yet know the (possible) answers to this question because the analysis has not yet been done. This collection has laid the foundations for such an analysis by starting to identify the range of possible factors and perspectives that would need to be included in just such a comparative analysis, but there is further work to be done.

This is particularly important as the developments continue to occur in DI itself, as well as in the blurring of boundaries between DI and other techniques such as *in vitro* fertilisation and in the development of newer techniques such as the micro manipulation of sperm. These developments not only emphasise further the dynamic nature of the field of assisted conception, they also help to raise questions about the simpler procedures, most notably whether the questions about any form of assisted conception are primarily concerned with the techniques themselves or with the social relationships that surround the use of such techniques? The chapters of this book reflect the primary concerns of social scientists in their consideration (predominantly though not solely) of the social relationships, rather than the techniques *per se*. Volumes such as that edited by Barratt and Cooke (1993) reflect the predominant (though not sole) concerns of practitioners with the technical aspects of DI. Clearly future work, not just on DI but on all aspects of assisted conception, will benefit from a closer collaboration of the two approaches, such that the social implications of the technical side of assisted conception can be analysed just as the technical implications of the social commentaries and recommendations can be fully appreciated. Developments such as the micro manipulation of poor quality sperm (HFEA Report 1993), do-it-yourself insemination and even sperm extraction from corpses (Freedland 1995) may seem to remove the need for DI in the future but the wider context of the technical and social implications of all these practices need to be investigated before it is clear under which circumstances one practice is preferable to the others. As the chapters in this book suggest, such an analysis takes time and has itself to be sufficiently dynamic to keep abreast of developments. However, this is not to suggest that no new developments be deployed until all the consequences of such developments be fully appreciated: that would only lead to stasis. Rather, it is simply to advise caution in assuming that all the problems of older techniques have been resolved simply because of the age of the technique or to assume that newer techniques will resolve the problems of older techniques simply through their newness. Instead, it is to urge practitioners, clinical scientists, social scientists and policy-makers at least to take account of the wider picture when developing/advocating the use of any technique.

Juengst (1993) provides one possible framework for gaining access to that wider picture, by outlining five questions to ask about any medical technology: they are as suitable to ask of assisted conception in general and donor insemination in particular as of any other intervention. A brief glance at these questions shows how contributors to this collection have helped to broaden the analysis of DI. The first question asks what the purposes of the technology are and points out that it is worth remembering that original purposes can have unintended consequences which may lead to a reevaluation of the original purpose. The chapters by Lasker, the Snowdens and by Haimes all provide answers to the question of the purpose of DI and examples of possible unintended consequences. The next question asks what value judgements are presumed by the technology, in terms of 'what should count as legitimate health problems and justifiable approaches to their resolution' (1993: 203). The chapters by Lasker, the Snowdens, Haimes, Daniels, Novaes and Edwards provide a range of answers to this question, including the possible disagreements that can occur in the field of fertility treatment. The third question asks who controls the technology, in terms of the relative strengths, and claims, of the clinical, contractual and commercial sectors. The chapters by Novaes and by Blank provide some pertinent insights in to how this question has been answered within the field of DI. The next question asks what external forces drive the technology, in terms of 'the multiple economic, social and political forces' (p. 204) that influence the dissemination and use of the intervention within the health care system. The chapters by Novaes, Edwards and Blank explore this issue and reveal a complex set of answers for DI. The final question asks what social risks arise from using the technology, in terms of the indirect consequences for the users and the wider society. The chapters by Lasker, the Snowdens, Haimes and by Daniels show that the social risks of DI are often unexpected but also pervasive in their effect on all parties directly involved.

An approach such as Juengst's is useful for a collection such as this since it serves as a contrast to the view presented here that DI can best be understood by fragmenting it into its effects on, and interpretations by, the different parties. We decided to take this approach since, amongst other reasons, it serves to emphasise the multidimensional context of DI practice, with a particular focus on the social relationships involved. Thus, we can see how each party interprets the practice and how each party regards the other parties involved in DI, to see which interests are shared and which are distinct. None the less, it is important to see that there are other approaches to painting the picture.

Part of the reason for the neglect of DI by social scientists has been the more general neglect of issues around reproduction in the social sciences, with a few notable exceptions. What is clear from this collection is that the study of assisted conception more generally and of DI in particular, reveals issues of much wider concern in sociological theory. The study of assisted conception contributes to the current central debates around risk, the concern with the globalisation of social experience, the postmodernist concerns with questioning the certainties of science and the authority of medicine, and to ideas and processes of social integration and exclusion. Equally it has to be acknowledged that the chapters in this collection have only skimmed the surface of other issues which the analysis of assisted conception has much to contribute to, such as the role of religion, issues of ethnicity, the debates around the body as a social construct and, finally, more detailed issues of masculinity. There is also much more to be said about the socio-legal, the moral/ethical and the philosophical debates around DI, which again have only been briefly touched upon in this collection, but we accept that those are more appropriately dealt with by others with more expertise in those academic disciplines.

In this volume we have built the foundations for further social science analyses of DI. Through conceptual analysis and empirical investigation we have begun to establish the nature of the social relationships that both constitute, and arise from, the practice of DI. We have also become clearer about the issues of policy and practice that require further attention and debate. Thus, a systematic study of DI, such as that presented in this book, has much to contribute, both to the pragmatic world of clinical practice and to the theoretical world of social science disciplines. However, we would be the last to claim that the social sciences alone can provide the final word on DI. Rather, we hope to have shown that there is a great potential for a dialogue between the social sciences and the other disciplines involved in DI, a dialogue to which all parties can contribute and from which all parties can benefit.

REFERENCES

Annas, G. and Elias, S. (1989) 'The treatment of infertility: legal and ethical concerns'. *Clinical Obstetrics and Gynaecology* 32(3): 614–21.
Barratt, C. and Cooke, I., eds. (1993) *Donor insemination.* Cambridge: Cambridge University Press.
Callahan, D. (1991) 'Opening the debate?' *The Milbank Quarterly* 69(1): 41–4.
Freedland, J. (1995) 'Sperm extracted from corpse in world first'. *The Guardian,* 21 January 1995.
Human Fertilisation and Embryology Authority (1993) *Second Annual Report.* London: HFEA.
Juengst, E. (1993) 'Developing and delivering new medical technologies: issues beyond access'. *Journal of Social Issues* 49(2): 201–10.

Index

For EU product safety concerns, contact us at Calle de José Abascal, 56–1°,
28003 Madrid, Spain or eugpsr@cambridge.org.

www.ingramcontent.com/pod-product-compliance
Ingram Content Group UK Ltd.
Pitfield, Milton Keynes, MK11 3LW, UK
UKHW010046140625
459647UK00012BB/1651